The
Emotional Diet

The Emotional Diet

How to Love Your Life More and Food Less

Bill Cashell

Fountain Hill Publishing

To my loving son Jeff
With faith, anything is possible

Contents

Introduction

We have heard that America is facing an epidemic. And the rest of the world is probably not far behind. For the first time in modern history, life expectancy may begin to shorten. After years of medical research and marvelous advances, we have become victims of our own excess. It has been estimated that over two-thirds of all Americans are overweight. Children are showing signs of adult onset diabetes in their early teens.

At any one time, more than 50 percent of women and 25 percent of men in America consider themselves on a diet. It seems like every day a new diet is hyped as the best way to lose weight. Television is bombarded with infomercials about exercise equipment that is guaranteed to make you look like a body builder or super model. Are any of these products really working? Every year we see more diets and products, and every year the population of America gets fatter.

Almost every magazine has an article about the magic solution to weight loss. We all talk about it, think about it, and keep looking for that magic pill that will allow us to eat all of the pasta and pie we want and still be slim and healthy.

We are all looking for the easy way to have our cake and eat it too. If you bought this book looking for another fad diet, you will not find it here. This is not a quick fix that will allow you to lose 10 pounds in one week.

There is no solution for turning cup-cakes into a sleek, sexy body. If you really want to make a permanent change in your weight, you have to make a permanent change in the way you eat. The key to making a permanent change in the way you eat is to change the way you feel about food. That is what this book is all about. Helping you change your whole attitude about how you eat, when you eat and especially why you eat. If you want to change your body, it starts with changing your mind.

1

For so many years, I tried to lose weight. I tried just about every diet that came out, always with the same result. Every diet would work for awhile, but I couldn't stick to it. Sometimes I would just get emotionally wound up and go on an eating binge for several days. No matter how much I ate, it was never enough to satisfy me. There were times when I ate so much I was miserable and I would still eat more. I knew it wasn't the food that I really craved. I was trying to fill some emotional need with food.

At times I would know what feeling it was. I might just be feeling sorry for myself or overwhelmed. There were other times when I just felt this overwhelming urge to eat and I didn't know why. I cursed myself for being so weak. Why couldn't I just use my will power? I knew I didn't need the food, especially bad food. To make it worse, I would get mad at myself and then punish myself by eating some high-fat, high-sugar food that I knew was bad for my body. It was almost like I was getting some strange pleasure in making myself miserable. The more I did it, the worse I felt. The worse I felt, the more I did it. I was in a vicious cycle and couldn't seem to break out. If it was so easy to just eat healthy food in small amounts, why couldn't I do it? What was wrong with me?

I spent several years trying to answer that question. I didn't like some of the answers I would get and my self-image and self-esteem just plummeted. You probably wouldn't have known it to talk to me, but when I talked to myself it was always negative. Why was it so easy for all of these other people and so hard for me? I admired them for their will power but at the same time I envied them and even despised the way they made it seem so easy. How could they leave food on their plate? How could they just pass up that plate of cookies as though they were made of play dough?

Most of all, I wanted to know why they could do it and I couldn't. I began to study psychology and how the mind works to find out what was driving me. The more I learned about the mind, the more fascinated I became. I was especially interested in techniques that seem to offer more rapid results like hypnosis and Neuro Linguistic Programming (NPL). The more I studied, the more I wanted to learn. I became certified in Hypnotherapy, NLP and EFT (Emotional Freedom Technique), all in an effort to create the changes that would finally let me take control of my eating.

The reason I was so driven was because I saw my weight as a cause of much of my unhappiness. I just knew that when I finally found a way to lose weight and keep it off, I would be happy. I somehow thought that it would be the answer to all of my problems. Once I could control my eating, I could take control of everything in my life. I would no longer be a procrastinator. People would love to be around me. I would finally be proud of myself and no longer feel like a failure. Maybe I could even learn to really love myself.

As I learned all of these techniques, I knew I had to also use them to help others. It was like I was going down a journey with many other people that were traveling the same road that I was. I was amazed to find out how much I had in common with others that struggled with their weight. So many issues that drive us to eat are things we are not even aware of. Many of us are still being haunted by past issues, some of which seem very trivial when we finally uncover and face them.

One big issue for me was the relationship I had with my father. To be more specific, it was the relationship I never really got to have. He was always too busy to spend time with me and criticized almost everything I did. It was his way of raising children that he had probably learned from his parents. He also had an issue with alcohol. Working with many people over the years, I have found this to be a very common theme with so many others. Another issue that shows up far more often than I would like to say is abuse of some type. So many people have faced physical, emotional or even sexual abuse in their past and they use food as a way to deal with repressed feelings. It is my belief that almost everyone has issues from their past that are causing them some type of emotional struggle. It is also my belief that most people have a lower self image of themselves than they deserve.

When I first started working with people, I knew that I could use hypnosis and other techniques to help people make changes. But somehow the title of "Hypnotherapist" kind of bothered me. I didn't know if I really wanted to be a therapist or felt that it was my role. I do have many good friends that are therapists and I love what they do. For me, it is all about change....rapid change. I quickly abandoned that term, although I still have my certifications on the wall to show people that I am qualified. When I work with people now, I tell them we are going to find out where they are, what is keeping them there, where they want to be and how to get there. If I feel someone has a deep psychological problem, I refer them to a qualified therapist.

In this book, I have put together the best techniques that I have found to help people break free from emotional eating and create the feelings of happiness that they deserve. You are about to go on a journey of self discovery. If you take the time to spend with yourself and go through the exercises, I think you will find the answers you are looking for. This book is not just for reading – it is for doing.

This journey will help you understand how food, emotions and so much else can affect our lives. You will learn how our minds were programmed to react the way we do toward food, and how we can reprogram them to react differently. To make changes in your life, you must have the desire to change, the knowledge to change and the willingness to follow through.

You don't change by just reading, you change by doing. This book will show you how. You probably have the desire, or you wouldn't have picked up this book. You will gain the knowledge as we go through.

The real success will depend on you. If you follow through and do all of the exercises, you will see changes happen easily and effortlessly. If you just read and don't bother to do the exercises, it means you really aren't serious about changing your life. This doesn't require sacrifice or great willpower. It does require the commitment to follow through for at least the next 30 days. You will find many techniques for change here. If you use them, you will find your life will change in so many ways.

Getting the Most from This Book

This book is probably different than any other weight loss book you have read. Most other books just tell you what to do, and then you have to battle with willpower. That's why most diets fail. This book is designed to show you how to do it. It is also interactive, so I will be with you every step of the way. The difference between a trim, healthy person and a heavy, unhealthy person is not ability and usually not knowledge.

There is not a heavy person in the world that doesn't know that broccoli is good for you and donuts are not. So what is the difference? How can one person eat healthy foods without a second thought while so many people struggle with their eating habits and their weight?

That's what this program is all about. If you have tried diet after diet, only to be frustrated by your lack of willpower, your time has come. This is not about pumping you up with motivation, it is about giving you the tools to change the way you feel about food and the way you feel about your life.

To that end, I believe that there are three keys to real success. You probably picked up this book because you wanted to lose weight. I will show you how to do that easily and effortlessly. However, losing weight is not enough. You could lose weight eating nothing but junk food if you cut down on the number of calories. That would not make you healthy. It would reduce your risk of many diseases, so that would be good, but not good enough. What we really want is total health.

If you follow some fad diet or a low carb diet, you would be able to reduce your weight but there are consequences to long-term diets like that. We also want to focus on emotional health because the way we feel emotionally affects the way we feel physically. It also affects what we eat, how we eat and even our digestive systems. People who feel good about their lives are much more likely to take care of themselves. So our three goals for this program are to be ***trim, healthy and happy***.

To create that type of life requires a lot of involvement on your part. This will be a journey that we will take together. I will guide you down the path, but you have to actually climb the mountain yourself. I'm sure you have heard about people saying how a book or a seminar or some other event literally changed their lives. If you are looking for that in this book, I hope you will find it. However, to find it, you will have to look past the book itself and into yourself.

The truth is that books, seminars and other events are not really life changing. The real changes come from the people that use the information and actually make the change. It may come suddenly in an "Ah Ha!" moment. The good news is that power exists within you. You have the ability to transform your body and your life into whatever you choose. I am not going to give you that ability. I am going to show you how to unleash the power that is already in you.

The television health channel has a program that chronicles people who have reached a point of obesity and then lost the weight permanently. There is one thing that all of these stories have in common. All of the people struggled with their weight, failing at diet after diet until they had an emotional change inside of themselves. For some, it could be the shame of an event where they were embarrassed by their weight. For others, it could be their family telling them they hoped they would be around to see their children grow up.

The change may have appeared to happen in an instant, because that is when the decision was made. For most of them, it took a long time to achieve the emotional power to make that commitment. Once that happens, the rest is almost automatic. I'll show you how to take yourself to that point of decision.

If you want this to be a life-changing event for you, it can be. The choice is yours. So many people are looking for that magic pill that will make them change so that they don't have to do it themselves.

The truth is that we are all living the life we choose. You may not like to admit it, if you are not happy with your life. It is so much easier to blame your parents or your genes or anything else that takes the blame off of you. It is like the people who want to sue the large hamburger restaurants for making them fat. No one advertises a burger and fries as diet food, but they want to blame someone else for their choices.

When you make someone else responsible for creating your problems, you are also giving them the responsibility of fixing them. Until you are ready to own your problems, your life will not change. The good news is, once you do own your problems, it is easy to find the solutions. Realize right now that you have the power to change virtually anything in your life. Decide that you are no longer willing to make excuses for anything in your life that is not the way you want it to be.

This book will help you get clear on making those decisions. For most people, making decisions about their life is like steering a boat by the wake. They are so focused on the turbulence behind them that they fail to see the smooth water ahead. They look back at where they have been and then head for the same water again. It is time to set your life course for new waters.

You will learn how to break free from your old habits and patterns, to break free from your old limiting beliefs and to boldly go where you have never gone before. This can be a life-changing journey for you, or it can be just another book that you start reading, hoping for that bolt of lightning to hit you. The choice is yours. The lightning is within you. All you have to do is harness it and you will never be the same again.

In some ways, you could compare this to a program for fixing your house. You could attend a workshop on home repair and get the tools and knowledge to fix all of the problems your house has. However, if you take the tools home and put them on the shelf, what happens to your house? That's right, it never gets fixed. After a period of time, it will even get worse.

In this program you will get the tools and the skills to use them. What you do from there, is up to you. If you put them on the shelf, your body and your life will stay the same or possibly decline a bit more over time. If you use the tools every day until you reach your goal, and then occasionally for maintenance, you will see the results you want.

Occasionally when I run into people who have attended my seminars, I hear one of two things. Either they applied these tools and created the results they wanted (and they are always very excited) or they are still the same and say how great the seminar was and that they intend to start using these techniques one of the days.

There is an old saying that "knowledge is power." The truth is, knowledge is only potential power. The power does not show up until you start to apply the knowledge.

In this book you will find several exercises that will ask you to do an assignment that requires some thought and writing down your results. If you just read past them, you will not find the answers that will help you create that life-changing experience.

All of the answers you need are within you. Only you can find them. I will show you where to look, but it is up to you to actually do the searching. What you find will help you create the roadmap to the trim, healthy, happy life that you have been searching for. Please take the time to give yourself this gift. Believe me, it will be worth it.

After working with hundreds of people with weight loss, I can tell you that it is different than most other issues. Phobias can often be released in a very short time. Smoking is different because you either smoke or you don't – there is no in between.

You have had a whole lifetime of creating associations to food. Think of it like a balance scale. Every time you eat unhealthy food and associate it to a feeling, you are adding more weight to that side of the scale. Every time you eat healthy foods and create new associations, you are putting weight on the other side of the scale. The more you repeat it, the more you create a shift inside of you.

Each of the techniques you will find here has been shown to work for most people. I have never found one that works every time for everyone, however some will come close. I have continued to add more techniques because everyone can find several that work for them. When you combine them, the power increases immensely.

Now, here is the good news – you will not have to starve yourself, feel deprived or battle with willpower. This program is all about changing your attitudes, habits and associations to food, exercise, health and what you are capable of.

The even better news is that you will find your life changing in so many ways. The techniques you learn here can be applied to almost anything you want to achieve in your life.

You have probably heard the expression, "Give someone a fish and you feed them for a day. Teach someone to fish and you feed them for a lifetime". The problem is that most people just want you to give them a fish. They don't want to take the time and effort to learn. I find this with weight issues as well. People say, "Just make me skinny" and I tell them, "First you have to learn what skinny people know. Then you can make the changes yourself". When you learn and use these techniques, you will be able to think and act like a thin person.

Now, here is the one thing you will have to remember. Even though it will not be difficult, it will take a commitment of time on your part. If you are willing to give yourself about 40 minutes every day for the next month, you will be rewarded with the life you want to create and the body you deserve.

Now is the time to get excited. Your journey is about to begin. Let's get started! For a personal introduction to this book, go the Emotional Diet web site at http://www.emotionaldiet.com/review.html.

At the end of each chapter, you will find an audio review on this web site. You can also download all of the worksheets for your exercises at http://www.emotionaldiet.com/downloads.html.

Chapter One

Why Diets Don't Work

"Insanity: doing the same thing over and over again and expecting different results".
- Albert Einstein -

I always start off my seminars by asking if anyone has ever been on a diet. Of course, every hand goes up. Then I ask if anyone has been on more than one diet. Again, every hand goes up. The reason they are here is because they have tried diet after diet without the long-term success that they want. Then I ask, "Would you like to have a diet that I guarantee will work as long as you don't have a problem with your metabolism?" I can see the excitement in their eyes as they prepare to receive the magic formula that will transform their lives. "Okay", I respond, "Here it is.........exercise more, eat less!"

This brings a few groans and a lot of smiles because they realize that it really is that simple. So why is it so hard to do? If all we need to do is put less food in our mouths and move more, why don't we do it? The reason is simple. We are not driven by logic we are driven by emotion.

We Are Not Driven by Logic - We Are Driven by Emotion

When an obese person has weight loss surgery, it does one thing. It restricts the amount of food they can put in their stomach by reducing the size of the stomach. That means anyone who has success with surgery can achieve the same result by reducing the amount of food they take in. It is as simple as that. We all have the ability to limit what we put in our body.

For most of my adult life, I intentionally gained two or three pounds every year until I was almost 250 pounds. I say I was intentionally overweight because I have never accidentally eaten anything. Everything I have put in my mouth has been to fill a need. Unfortunately, that need is usually emotional and not physical.

That is why surgery is not the answer. Recently on a television documentary, the feature was about a teenage girl from Houston who weighed 368 pounds. The point of the program was that teenage obesity is becoming a big problem and the diseases associated with being overweight are showing up at a younger age.

The surgery they were performing is called gastric bypass. It had only been performed on a few teenagers before. The concern was that they didn't know what effect this could have on a body that had not finished growing. The greater concern was that the poor girl would not live to see twenty if her weight was not reduced.

They followed her before, during and after the surgery to record how she was handling each step. She was anxious to have the surgery because she had been unable to control her eating on her own. There was also some fear of creating this change in her life.

The surgery went well with no complications. I should mention that this is considered major surgery, and there are some risks involved. This is not a foolproof procedure, and you should be aware that the results are not always as good as they appear.

The results are also not always as permanent as people would believe. The stomach has the ability to stretch, and often the people who have this procedure will reach a certain point and start gaining weight back. In fact, it is not unusual for them to gain most or all of the weight they have lost from the surgery. This will certainly make many people think twice about rushing into it.

Several weeks after the surgery, the young girl was interviewed to see how she was faring. On the scale, the news was good. She had lost 38 pounds already.

You would think that she would be thrilled, but it was just the opposite. In her own words, she felt like "she had lost her best friend". She went into a period of deep depression and stopped taking her vitamins. These were essential because the small amount of food that she was able to consume could not supply enough nutrients. She had to be hospitalized until she was stable enough to resume her normal life. She still continued to struggle with the emotional need that food had given her, a need that was now missing.

One of her doctors was interviewed about this factor and he said, "This is the problem that she will probably struggle with all of her life". That is not a very bright future. They were trying to fix the result without addressing the cause. Perhaps if they had resolved her emotional needs, she wouldn't have needed the surgery.

Is this how you feel about food? Do you have some emotional connections that you are afraid to let go of? Most of us do. That is why I feel the doctors really missed the mark on this. They were trying to fix the problem by treating the condition. Unfortunately, they didn't address the cause of the problem, which will cause it to return if not resolved.

That is what this book is all about. It is about helping you find out what is causing your emotional eating and giving you the tools to have a happier, more fulfilling life without the need for food as a constant companion.

The Easiest Way to Gain Weight is Yo-Yo Dieting

This book is not going to give you another diet. I really don't believe in diets. In fact, the easiest way to gain weight is yo-yo dieting. Studies show that most people who go on a diet will gain back all of the weight they lost plus an additional two pounds. To make matters worse, this usually results in adding to the fat content in your body.

When you lose weight quickly, your body will often start by burning the glucose that is immediately available and then start burning the fat reserves. Unfortunately, your body may also start breaking down protein as well, reducing your muscle mass. When you gain weight back quickly, it is usually stored as fat. That means that the combination of fast weight loss and fast weight gain can increase the fat ratio in your body.

13

Lose 7 Pounds in 7 Days

One problem is that most people are impatient when it comes to weight loss. We all want to lose 20 pounds by tomorrow. That is why it is so easy to get sucked into the advertisements that promise to help you "lose 7 pounds in 7 days". Let's take just a minute and look at that, because it is really easy to lose 7 pounds in 7 days.

We know that it takes about 3500 calories to make a pound of body weight. To gain another pound, you would have to take in 3500 more calories than you burn up. To lose one pound, you would have to burn up 3500 more calories than you consume.

Let's say that a person needs 2500 calories to maintain their current body weight. They go on a diet that reduces their intake by 1000 calories so they are now taking in 1500 calories. The first thing that often happens is your body retains less water, so you may lose two pounds of water weight the first week.

Most people have somewhere between 5 and 15 pounds of undigested food in their intestines at any given time, especially if you eat a lot of meat or little fiber. When you cut back drastically, your body will eliminate more waste than you put in. That may give you another three pounds. By cutting back 1000 calories per day, you are burning an extra 7000 calories per week, which is the equivalent of two pounds of actual body mass.

On the scale, you have "lost" seven pounds. You could gain five of those back the first day you resume normal eating.

What I'm going to ask you to consider now is the idea of losing the weight slowly at the rate of about one pound per week or even less. The problem most people have with losing weight slowly is that they want instant results.

Now, here is the good news. You can have those instant results. If you change the type of food you are eating to a healthy diet, you will feel the difference in 24 hours. That's right! By this time tomorrow you can have more energy, more vitality and just feel better all around. How does that sound?

I know what you are thinking. You want to feel good, but you also want to lose the weight quickly. The truth is, you can do that without having to drop a pound every day. Let me use the example I use in my seminars. I bring a pound of bacon and pass it around for everyone to see and feel. If you have a pound of bacon in your house, go look at it now. If not, look at it the next time you go to the grocery store. What you will notice is that most bacon is 75 to 80 percent fat.

Now, before we go any further, let me say a few words about bacon. This is positively one of the worst foods you can put into your body. As I mentioned, bacon is about ¾ pure fat. For some odd reason, we seem to have this illusion that if we fry it up until it turns brown, it will become meat. It is not meat! It is brown fat!

To make it worse, bacon contains a preservative called sodium nitrite, which has been linked to cancer. When you fry it in its own grease, it releases cancer-causing nitrates. So you are eating fried fat that causes cancer.

Let me ask you this: would you take a slab of fat and just start eating it?

Probably not.

Would you take a slab of fat and fry it and then eat it?

Probably not.

Then why would you eat a slab of fried fat that has just a little bit of meat running through it? What is really interesting is that most people who eat bacon will be very careful to cut all of the excess fat off the steak they eat. Does that make sense?

Of course it doesn't when you think about it. It is just one of those things we have been conditioned to eat. You actually can get bacon without all of the fat. It's called ham. Another substitute would be Canadian bacon. There are other substitutes that are much healthier. We'll get more into that later.

Let's get back to our visual of the pound of bacon. By the way, the pound of bacon I use for demonstrations is particularly high in fat and it looks like it is almost pure fat. When people pass it around, they get the experience of actually seeing and feeling a pound of fat. Then I ask if they would like to peel that much fat off of their bodies by this time next week. The answer is always yes. A pound of thick sliced bacon usually has about 14 slices in it.

If you cut back only 250 calories per day, it is equal to peeling a thick slice of bacon from your body. When you think of a pat of butter having 100 calories, it is pretty easy to cut back 250 calories per day. If you increase your activity level by only 250 calories per day, that is equal to pulling another strip of bacon from your body.

Avoid cutting back on your calorie intake too much. When you do, your body will slow down your metabolism because it wants to avoid starvation.

If you are looking for quick results, you can have it. By this time tomorrow, you can have more energy, more vitality and have two strips of fat the size of thick bacon gone from your body!

That should be your goal every day. To cut back enough calories to peel off one strip of bacon and increase your physical activity enough to peel off another strip of bacon. Every time you look at some cake or pie or other unhealthy fattening food, imagine that eating it will put two strips of bacon back on your body.

Because that is what really happens. Any unhealthy food you eat will probably end up as excess fat on your body. If you feel you must have it to feed an emotional urge, have a smaller piece and only put one strip of bacon on your body. That way, if you peel off two strips, you are still reducing your body fat.

Even 100 calories is enough to make a difference. That would still be equal to one half strip of normal bacon everyday!

That is your new goal – to reduce your body fat. Forget about your weight and focus on the fat. That is what you really want to get rid of.

Why You Choose Food Instead of Change

Why is it so easy to eat this food that you know is unhealthy and you know will make you fat? The reason is, we respond to what is most immediate. When the phone rings, we stop important tasks to answer it because it is immediate. We don't know if it is important, but it is right there ringing at this very minute.

This is what happens in your mind when you see the food in front of you; it is there right now. When you think of being trim and healthy, it is somewhere in the future. You will usually go for what is most immediate. Then you tell yourself (and everyone around you) I'll get back to healthy eating tomorrow (or that line we have all used – I'll start my diet Monday).

Here is how you can take control right now:

Imagine that there are two doors in front of you leading to your immediate future.

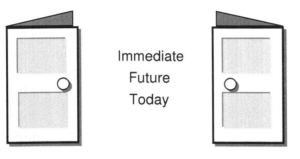

Junk Food   **Healthy Body**

If you walk through the one on the left, you can eat the unhealthy food you desire right now.

If you walk through the one on the right, you will immediately have the body you desire right now.

You already know you can't have both, so you have to make a choice. When both choices are immediate, it makes the decision pretty easy. When I ask this question, people always choose the healthy body. That is why it is so important to remember that your body is changing today, not next year, or next month or even next week.

You will either peel off that strip of fat today or put it back on. Keep that image of the fat strips of bacon in your mind every time you eat. Whatever door you feel is most immediate is the one you will be drawn toward. Your future is being created right now. *Everything you eat today will determine how you look and feel tomorrow.*

You Might Want to Hide Your Scale

Some people have an obsession with their weight. They will weigh themselves every day and sometimes several times each day. There are three things that can happen when you get on the scale, and all three can cause problems. The first is that your weight has gone down. This can get you really excited. You may even jump up and down screaming, "Yes! I did it!" Then you feel this rush of excitement and this wonderful feeling that you should reward yourself. You decide that since you have done so well, you can now have ice cream and pizza. There goes your diet!

The second result is that your weight is still the same. After depriving yourself all day, nothing has changed. You know in your mind that it sometimes takes a little time for your weight to adjust, but right now that doesn't matter. You were good all day and you want to see the results of your struggle right now. You get discouraged and go right for the ice cream. So much for the diet!

The third result is that your weight actually went up. How can that be? You were so good all day and you want that scale to tell you that it was worth it. But now, it sits there laughing at you, teasing you like this is some cruel joke. You throw your hands up and say, "What's the use!" and head right for the cookie jar. You completely ignore the fact that your body may be retaining water. The next day you jump on the scale expecting the worst from those cookies and you are down a pound. "That's it!" you scream, "I just need to eat more cookies!"

It's Not Your Weight, It's Your Fat

The two measurements that are most important are your waist measurement and your blood pressure. Being overweight will make you feel uncomfortable,

18

but excess weight around your midsection and high blood pressure will kill you. If you are fortunate enough to carry your weight all over your body (you may not consider that fortunate, but bear with me) it is much healthier for you. The fat around your vital organs can be the most dangerous place to store it. If you want to measure something, measure your waist and your blood pressure. Also remember that muscle weighs more than fat. You could reduce your size and actually gain "weight" if you build muscle. This is a good thing!

What You Really Need to Change is Not Your Weight

What if I could wave a magic wand over you and you would be at your perfect weight? Would that make you happy? Sure it would. Now, here's the rest of the question. If you kept the same behavior you have now, where would you be in six months? Most people will say they would be right back where they are now.

This leads us to the single most important point in this book: What you really need to change is not your weight. What you really need to change is your behavior.

Your current weight is a result of your current behavior. Unfortunately, most diets are aimed at changing the result. That makes dieting a short-term goal. When you reach your goal weight, you can't wait to go out and eat all of those foods you have been craving. Before long, your weight is creeping up so...back on the diet.

This becomes a never-ending battle because you are focused on changing the result and you haven't changed the cause. Since your current weight is a result of your current behavior, all you have to do is change your behavior and your weight will automatically change. And this way it will become a permanent change so that you never have to diet again.

From now on, you are going to focus on changing your behavior. No more diets. Change your behavior and your weight will take care of itself.

Diets are self-defeating and they are a temporary goal. Forget your scale and forget your weight. For the next thirty days, you are going to ignore any thought of dieting and work on your mind and your emotions. Say good-bye to diets because you are now taking control of your behavior. Once you learn to do this, you will see changes happening in every part of your life. You are going to be awesome!

Your current weight is a result of your current behavior.
What you really need to change is NOT your weight.
What you really need to change is your behavior.

Your Mind Does Not Respond Well to a Negative Goal

One of the reasons people fail on diets is because a diet is a negative goal. Let me give you an example by asking a few questions.

Would you like to lose some money? Of course not!

Would you like to lose some time? Heck no!

Would you like to lose some of your close friends? No, you love your friends.

Would you like to lose weight? Hmmm…well, yes I would!

Do you see what is happening? At a conscious level, we say we want to "lose weight". At a subconscious level, we have been programmed throughout our lives to not "lose" anything. We don't want to lose any possessions, we don't want to lose our minds, and we don't even want to lose at card games.

In sports, there are winners and losers. We don't want to be a loser. Since this is happening at a subconscious level, we have this internal battle going on between what we think we want and what is really driving us.

Remember, we are driven by our emotions and those are stored in the subconscious mind. The whole idea of losing weight and depriving yourself goes against your internal programming. Your mind does not respond well to a negative goal.

Now it is time to redirect your thoughts and create a goal that will pull you to success.

You Are Drawn Toward Whatever You Focus On

When you go on a diet, what do you think about? Food, of course! Since we are drawn toward whatever we think about, you have just created a stronger desire for what you are trying to avoid. Now you are trying to use willpower to control your behavior, but you have directed your subconscious mind toward food. If you hold on to your willpower, you feel like you have deprived yourself. If the desire wins out, you feel like a failure because you don't have enough willpower.

Remember this: *you are drawn toward whatever you focus on.* When you focus on what you don't want, you get more of it. You can't become thin by thinking about how fat you are or obsessing about food. Most of the time we focus on what we don't want! That is a recipe for automatic failure.

The word "don't" is really kind of a funny word. It is a contraction made up of two opposing words. The first part "do" means that something will happen. The second part "not" means that nothing will happen. Our minds actually think in images, even if you think you are not a visual person. Since there is no way to create an image of "don't", our minds tend to bypass it.

Let me give you an example. Right now, don't think of a pizza. What are you thinking of? I know, you are thinking of a pizza. The reason is, to not think of a pizza you have to first think of what you don't want to think about.

Confusing? Let's take an example. If you have children or have been around children, you have probably had something like this happen. You tell the kids, "Don't eat the cookies before dinner". Five minutes later they are covered in cookie crumbs. You get angry and tell them they didn't listen to you.

21

The fact is, they listened perfectly. When you said, "Don't eat the cookies before dinner", what kind of image does that create? That's right! It creates an image of eating the cookies before dinner. Since we are drawn toward whatever we focus on, you have just created a desire to eat the cookies before dinner.

If you want to have success, you have to give yourself a positive goal of what you want instead of what you don't want. In the case of the cookies, you might say "Save the cookies until after dinner". Notice the new image it creates?

Another problem with negative goals is, when you tell yourself what you don't want, you have no direction of what you do want. Let me give you an example.

Suppose you want to go on a vacation and you said "I don't want to go to Milwaukee on my vacation". Where will you end up? You have said where you don't want to go, but there is no direction to guide you to where you do want to go.

Since you have said where you "don't" want to go, where are you thinking of? Probably Milwaukee. Remember, we are drawn toward whatever we think of.

Now, let's put that in terms of our weight. If you said, "I don't want to be fat anymore", what are you setting yourself up to be? You know the answer to that one.

You will never become thin by thinking about how fat you are. You need to give your mind the direction of what you really want. And what you really want is to be trim and healthy. Notice I didn't just say trim or thin. You could be at the ideal weight you want to be by eating junk food if you ate a small amount, but would you be healthy? I'm sure you've seen people like that who are thin but look like they could drop over at any minute. So your new focus is to be trim and healthy.

Everything you want to achieve in life goes through stages. You start with a dream of what you want to have or be. The more you think about that dream, the stronger your desire becomes. If you really hold on to that desire with passion and belief, it becomes an intention.

You've dreamed about changing your life for a long time. You have at least a strong enough desire to read this book. Now we want to make that desire even stronger. We will also create the necessary beliefs to make your dream come true. It is time for that dream to become an intention. You are now going to become the person you intend to be. The key to doing all of this is to identify with clarity, what you will look like, feel like, act like and believe. Once you do all of that, you are on the journey to becoming that person.

Let's get started programming that computer in your head right now. You can do this with your eyes open or closed, whatever works best for you.

Right now, imagine the perfect person you intend to be.

Notice how good you look and feel.

Notice how much energy and vitality you have.

Notice how people compliment you on how good you look.

Notice how good you feel about yourself.

Notice how you walk with a feeling of confidence and joy.

Notice how you enjoy healthy foods and pass up those unhealthy foods.

Notice how you look forward to exercise because it makes you feel so energized.

The more you focus on the person you want to become, the more your subconscious mind will direct your behavior to match that image. After awhile, you will find that you avoid unhealthy food and large quantities because your subconscious minds says, "That does not match that internal image and feeling I have of myself".

Everything you want to create in your life starts in your mind. Start every day with this exercise of imagining the perfect you that you intend to be. Make it as vivid and real as you can. Repeat it several times throughout the day and you will begin to notice that your behavior will start to change. You will be drawn toward what you focus on, which is being trim and healthy.

You are drawn toward whatever you focus on.
You will never be trim and healthy if you focus on how fat you are.
Focus on what you want and you will attract it.

Create a Blueprint for Your Future

You now have a way to direct your mind toward your new goal every morning. Now it is time to really get crystal clear on what you want. Right now, write down exactly what your life is going to be like. Be sure to write your life script as though it has already happened. Describe how you look and feel in detail. Write down how you act and react to every situation you can think of. Forget about how you might have acted in the past.

This is your blueprint for your new actions. If you don't want to write in the book, take out a sheet of paper and write everything that comes to mind. Keep writing until you have a clear vision of how you have chosen to live.

Please take the time to do this exercise. Studies have shown that when you write down what you want and make it crystal clear, you will achieve 80% of what you write. Write with passion and feeling to bring it to life.

My Blueprint for Success

<u>Describe in detail the new you.</u> What do you look like? What do you wear? What size are your clothes? How do you feel?

Examples: I now wear size _____ dress / pants.
   I feel so good when I pass up donuts.
   I enjoy thinking about my great life instead of food.

_____
_____
_____
_____
_____
_____
_____
_____
_____
_____
_____
_____

<u>Describe your behavior</u>. What do you do? What do you eat? How do you feel?

_____
_____
_____
_____
_____
_____
_____
_____

Now, mark this page or save the paper you wrote this exercise on. You can download a printable copy of this page at http://www.emotionaldiet.com/downloads.html.

Every morning you are going to imagine being the person you have chosen to become. Start by reading the description you just finished writing. This will make it consistent and create the same experience every time. After you read your script, close your eyes and imagine going through your day this way. The more you repeat it, the more it becomes a part of you.

Identify your new beliefs. Now you have a clear picture of the person you intend to be. This is obviously different from the person you have been in the past. One of the things that is different between your behavior and the behavior of people that are trim and healthy are your beliefs about what you can and can't do, and the forces that drive your behavior. To become the person you intend to be, you have to change your limiting beliefs to empowering beliefs. Think about what you would have to believe about yourself, your associations with food, the things that drive your behavior and anything else that you would have to believe to be this person.

I would have to believe:

_____

_____

_____

_____

_____

_____

_____

_____

_____

_____

_____

_____

_____

_____

_____

_____

If these beliefs seem foreign to you right now, that is great. That means you are starting to see what you need to change to draw you toward your goals. If you need to think about this a little bit, that is all right. You may even want to talk to some people that are trim and healthy and find out what they believe. Please be sure to complete these exercises. In a later chapter we will cover how you can integrate these beliefs into your nervous system.

Seeing is believing. Once you start seeing yourself as the person you intend to be, you will start to become that person. Decide how you want your life to be and say it out loud or write it down and read it every day as you imagine yourself as that person. Here are some suggestions that you can use right now to see yourself as already being that person:

I see myself with a trim and healthy body that is just perfect for me.

I see myself as the happy, loving person I was meant to be.

I see myself enjoying healthy foods in just the right amounts.

I see myself free of the negative feelings and emotions that held me back.

I see myself loving and being loved unconditionally.

I see myself feeling energetic, inspired and filled with enthusiasm.

I see myself poised and confident, filled with the belief that I am already successful.

I see myself feeling happy being me, knowing that I am a special person.

I see myself enjoying happiness every day, finding joy in everything I do.

Write down any of your own statements that you feel are right for you.

_____

_____

_____

_____

_____

_____

Shift Your Thinking

Just before the start of one of my seminars, a woman came up to me and asked, "Are you going to make me not like cookies?" I looked back at her and replied, "I'm not going to make you do anything, but it sounds like you have an issue with cookies. What's going on?"

"Well", she said, "I will buy a package of cookies and open them and then I eat the whole package".

"What do you want to do?" I asked.

"I want to be able to open the package and just eat a few", she said.

"All right", I answered, "We can probably do that, but let me ask you one question. How would it be if you lost your desire for cookies?"

Suddenly her face got this blank stare and she didn't say a word. The idea of giving up cookies had never crossed her mind. I think that is one problem that most of us face. We have associated pleasure with certain foods and we don't want to give them up.

Everyone is looking for that magic pill that will let us eat all of the junk food and comfort food we want and still be trim and healthy. It's time to shift your thinking on that. It will not happen. Science may come up with a pill that will suppress our appetites or block the fat or even let us eat junk food and stay thin. But you will never be healthy eating junk food. Eating cookies and taking a vitamin does not give you good nutrition. Your body needs good nutrition to stay healthy and to have the energy and vitality to really enjoy life on your terms.

Right now, start thinking about the possibility of enjoying healthy foods and breaking the emotional ties to the unhealthy foods. You are going to learn how to release those associations to unhealthy foods and create a desire for the foods that nourish your body and bring good health. The key word is freedom. You will be free of the bonds that hold you back from being the person you were meant to be. It is time to shift your thinking and get excited.

The Vicious Cycle of Emotional Eating

One problem we create is the vicious cycle of emotional eating. Imagine that you are about to go home from work and your boss comes in and says, "I'm sorry, some emergency has come up and you are going to have to work late tonight". You tell your boss that you have plans to go out with friends tonight to see a show and you already have the tickets. Unfortunately, you are the only one that can handle this matter, so you are stuck. All kinds of emotions run through your mind. You are angry because you can't join your friends and you had plans. You are frustrated because you have to work late. You look over at your coworker's desk and you see a big bowl of M&Ms. Even though you have stuck to your diet all day, you reach over and grab a big handful. Of course, you can't eat only one. That would just be an M. They travel in packs! That's why they call them M&Ms. One handful leads to another until you have finished the entire bowl. Now you really feel bad because you are still stuck at work and you have just blown your diet.

What do you say to yourself? You know what you say. You ask yourself, "Why did I do that?" Then you beat yourself up for your behavior and you feel like a failure. This really puts a dent in your self-esteem. To make it worse, it starts a new behavior of conditioned response. You now have a trigger that says the next time you feel that feeling of frustration; you reach for M&Ms or some other type of chocolate. The next time you are in this situation, you are very likely to resort to the same behavior without even thinking. The more you repeat this behavior, the more it becomes a habit. You beat yourself more each time and your self-esteem continues to go down as you tell yourself how weak you are. Every time you do that, you are reinforcing the same behavior and feeling bad about it. In the next chapter, we will see how you can easily break out of this cycle. For now, just realize that you are doing it and that you can change.

Make Your Happiness Unconditional

One mistake that so many people make is that they make their happiness conditional and they usually don't even know they are doing it. You hear people all the time saying things like, "When I lose 30 pounds, then I'll be happy" or "When I get a better job, then I'll be happy" or "When I get into a great relationship, then I'll be happy". The list goes on and on.

The problem is that when you make a statement like that, you are basically telling yourself that you will have to be unhappy until that happens. You probably don't mean it that way, but that is how the subconscious part of your mind is hearing it. And what happens if you never lose those 30 pounds, or get that better job, or get into that great relationship?

Does that mean you can never be happy? It's really up to you.

Have you ever been driving on a busy street and had someone cut right in front of you? Doesn't that make you mad? And if you don't drive, think of some similar experience when someone else makes you angry. Maybe it's because someone forgot your birthday or didn't do what you expected them to do. I think we have all had experiences like that.

Now, let me ask this question. Do you have to get mad? Is it required? The reality is that this is a choice we make. If someone cuts you off in traffic and you say they made you mad, you are letting them push your buttons. You are giving them control of your emotions. It's like saying that you don't have any choice in the matter. This leads to an even bigger problem. When you say that someone made you mad, you are now giving them responsibility to make you happy. If it's the driver that cut in front of you, the only way you will be happy is if they get a ticket. If it's the person that missed your birthday, they are going to have to apologize to you and make it up to you before you are happy.

When your happiness depends on someone or something else, you have no control of when or even if you will be happy. The truth is, you don't have to let someone else dictate your happiness. How you feel about every experience in your life is based on how you react to it. If someone cuts in front of you, can you choose to be happy? Of course you can. You could even laugh about it if you want. You could be happy that you are not riding with them or be happy that you didn't have an accident. How about the friend that forgot your birthday? You could be happy that you have a friend that you feel that close to. You could be happy that you had another birthday. As Abraham Lincoln once said, "Most people are about as happy as they make up their mind to be". It's time to make up your mind to be happy.

So what does that have to do with your weight and eating habits? One of the most common triggers for eating is a negative emotion. Have you ever turned to food when you were angry or frustrated or stressed? Remember the vicious cycle of emotional eating? Think how much better you would act if you were happy almost all of the time. There would be no need to turn to food to make you feel good because you already feel good. Studies show that it is easier for people to lose weight when they are happy. There is also an added health benefit to this. When you feel happy, your body releases chemicals called endorphins that make you feel good. These will also boost your immune system, helping your body recover from illness and improve your general health.

The Mind/Body Connection - You Can Be Happy Right Now

The idea of choosing to be happy may be a foreign idea at first, so we are going to do some exercises that will help you feel happy at any time. As I just mentioned, it's not what happens to you that creates a feeling, it is how you choose to respond to it. Right now, think about something in your life that makes you happy. It may be a person that you know or have known, it could be a place you've been that inspires you or brings back great memories, or it could be the memory of a happy time that you experienced. Now, close your eyes and really connect with that experience. See the sights, hear the sounds and really allow yourself to connect with that feeling. Any time you want to feel happy, all you have to do is come back to this experience and feeling. We all have the ability to focus on something that makes us happy if we choose. Remember this experience because we will use it again later to anchor these great feelings and bring them back instantly.

Let's look at another way to feel happy. Your mind and body are both connected to your nervous system. That means if you change what your mind is focused on, it will affect your body. Remember, when you focus on a pleasant experience like you just did, it will cause your body to release those "feel good" chemicals called endorphins. You will find that you are much more likely to avoid emotional eating when you feel good.

If you did this exercise effectively, you have already experienced how good it feels. You can also do it in reverse. Right now, think of something that makes you feel sad or depressed. You probably don't want to make it too serious, just something that might bother you a little bit. Think about how your posture would normally be if you felt bad. You would probably be slouched down, eyes down with shallow breathing. Now, as you are thinking of what makes you feel bad, stand up straight with a strong posture, and look up toward the ceiling and smile as big as you can. If someone is watching, it will just make him or her wonder what you are up to. Notice how you are not able to keep feeling bad when you do this? The reason is because your body is sending messages to your nervous system that you feel good. Since your mind is also connected to your nervous system, it receives the same message that you feel good. The fastest way to feel good is to change your body and your posture. If you smile and hold on to a positive posture, your body will override other negative feelings and you will feel good right away.

Now, let's see how you can use this to help you move toward your goal. You already have a blueprint for your future that describes the person you have chosen to become. Every morning you are going to read this and imagine it has already happened and that you are that person. You will find it is much easier to create a resourceful attitude if you feel positive about your life. Start every morning by thinking about what is good in your life. Think of what you are grateful for. Remember the experiences that have shaped you and helped you learn. Take a moment every morning to do this to create that positive emotional state before you use your blueprint for success.

Program Yourself for Success Every Day

Every morning, take a few minutes to just relax your mind and your body. Let all of the tension drift out of your body as you allow yourself to go into a meditative state. When thoughts come into your mind, just let them go and focus on your breathing. You may want to just repeat the word "relax" to yourself silently, over and over until your mind is clear of other thoughts. Now, think of what you are grateful for. It can be anything. It may just be the fact that you are alive. If you say you don't have anything to be grateful for, you are using your mind to focus on what is wrong instead of what is right. Realize that this is a choice and that you can choose to think of what is good in your life. Then, think of what you have to be happy about. It may be past experiences or people you have known. Take as long as you need to really feel good about your life.

Now, pick up your blueprint for your future and read it slowly aloud. As you do, allow the meaning of the words to come to life. Then, close your eyes and imagine that you have already achieved your desires. Notice how your behavior has changed to match the person you have chosen to be. Notice how good it feels to be that person. Imagine yourself going through the day eating only healthy foods and enjoying high energy. Notice how you pass up unhealthy foods without any desire for them. Notice how good you feel about yourself. Notice how people admire you for the way you look and your self-control. Feel how strong your body has become by eating the foods that nourish it.

Imagine yourself putting more exercise in your day by walking more and even taking a few minutes to give yourself the gift of regular exercise. Notice how you actually look forward to exercise because it is part of your life now and it makes you feel good. Now, notice how great it feels to be the person you always wanted to be. Connect those good feeling to your new behavior because you deserve to have those good feelings about this wonderful life you have chosen. Hold on to that feeling for as long as you like. Slowly open your eyes and smile, knowing that you are now creating your own life the way you want it to be.

Remember, we said we are drawn toward whatever we focus on. If you focus on food, you create a desire for food. If you focus on being trim and healthy, you create a desire to be trim and healthy. Several times during the day, bring back that image and the feelings of the perfect you; the person you have chosen to become. The more you reinforce this image, the more it becomes part of who you are.

33

After a short time you will notice that eating junk food does not match the image you have given your mind. Before long, your subconscious will start rejecting junk food because it does not match the image you have created for yourself. You don't have to use willpower because you will be drawn toward whatever you focus on and your desire to be trim and healthy will guide your behavior.

Daily Assignment

Every morning, take 5 minutes and program yourself for success. Start by thinking about what you have to be grateful for. Think of your friends, family, people in your life, good things that have happened to you, possibilities for the future, even the fact that you are alive. Everyone has something to be thankful for. When you think about what is good in your life, you become more resourceful and you get more of what you think of.

Look at your blueprint for success to have a clear picture of what you are creating. Use your powerful imagination to create your new behavior and become the person you choose to be. Imagine yourself having already reached your goal, going through your day with confidence and ease. The life you create in your mind becomes the life you live.

You can download a 6 ½ minute mp3 file for listening before reading your blueprint at http://www.emotionaldiet.com/downloads.html.

We are all living the life we choose.
If you want your life to change, the choice must come from you.

For a review of Chapter 1 go to
http://www.emotionaldiet.com/review.html.

Chapter Two

Your Emotional Self

"When dealing with people, remember you are not dealing with creatures of logic, but creatures of emotion". ~Dale Carnegie

I've often heard sales people say that customers buy with emotion and justify with facts. We all have that need to justify our actions whenever we can. On those occasions when we find it hard to see any logical reason for eating that jelly donut, we feel like we are not in control of our actions. It's like some invisible force is guiding us to do something we know is wrong but we just can't stop. As we've already said, we are not driven by logic, we are driven by emotion. The answer is not to create some internal struggle using willpower, which will ultimately fail. The answer is to make our emotions work for us.

What If You Had No Emotions?

You may or may not be familiar with the split hemisphere theory of the brain. Basically, the right side of your brain is the creative, emotional part of the brain and the left side is the logical, reasoning side of the brain. We often refer to logical thinkers as "left-brained" and creative, emotional people as "right-brained". Actually, very few people are totally one or the other. The two hemispheres are connected by a bundle of nerves called the corpus callosum, which allows the two sides to communicate with each other and work as one unit.

Several years ago, I watched a program about a man who had a serious brain injury which resulted in having part of his brain removed. In this case, all of the damage was done to the right side of the brain. This man was still able to function and lead a somewhat normal life. He was still able to reason and think, much like you and me. What was different for him was that he had no emotions. He didn't have to worry about emotional eating because he had no attachment to food. For him, food was strictly something for nourishment. Before you start calling your doctor to schedule a lobotomy, you should realize that he had absolutely no pleasure from the food he did eat. In fact, nothing gave him pleasure because that is an emotion. He was never happy, never sad, never excited, never bored, he just went through life thinking and doing everything out of necessity. There was no reason to watch a movie or spend time with family and friends, because it didn't serve any practical purpose. This man was trim and healthy, but it was an awful price to pay. Besides that, my guess is that the main reason you would like to be trim and healthy is because it would feel good. There you go, trying to fill an emotional need again.

It has been my experience that people who are left-brain dominant, usually have an easier time sticking to a diet and just ignoring food. You probably don't fall in that category or you wouldn't be reading this book right now. Being very emotionally driven can feel like a curse when you are trying to stick to that diet without lasting success. The good news is that people who are emotionally driven are able to create changes easily using the methods in this book.

Internal or External - That is the Question

How you feel at any given time is determined by the way you are managing your emotional states. Humans experience many different emotions, often changing from one to another very quickly. Some of these are positive like happiness, love, confidence, and passion while others can feel negative such as fear, sadness, pain, worry, boredom, loneliness, hate and anger.

It is human nature to move toward things that give us pleasure and away from anything that gives us pain. That is why so many people use food to change the way they feel. When something happens that makes them feel one of these negative feelings, they reach for a box of cookies to change the way they feel. The problem is, that only gives them a temporary change and does not do anything to address the real issue. In fact, it usually makes them feel bad for eating because it wasn't the food they really wanted, it was the feeling they thought the food would give them.

So, what are emotions for? Why do we need these negative feelings? Often when you feel one of these feelings, it is a sign that something is not right in your life. Think of your feelings like the gauges or lights on the dashboard of your car. If your electrical system is malfunctioning, a warning light comes on to let you know there is a problem. Would you try to fix the problem by putting more gas in the car? Of course not! But haven't you done that to yourself in the past? You feel some negative feeling and you try to fix it by putting more food in your body. That does not do anything to address the cause of the feeling, and as long as that feeling is there, you are likely to keep putting food in your body to change the way you feel.

Realize that these negative feelings are not really bad. They are warning lights, just like in your car, telling you that something is not right. See this as an opportunity to "fix" the problems in your life. You don't have to live that way anymore.

Emotions are complex states which have both internal and external representations. Generally, an emotion is a response to something. Most emotions are learned and become a conditioned response. Most people feel like they have no control over their emotions. When they are confronted by some external stimulus, they go straight to a particular emotion and may even remain in that emotion for a period of time.

It is important to realize that it is not what happens to you that "makes" you feel a certain way. It is the way you internalize and react to it that creates the feeling. What makes one person happy may make another person sad. The ways that people internally and externally represent an emotion can differ dramatically.

The Conditioned Response

Most of your actions are the result of previous experiences. When you do something in response to any given situation, you are creating a pattern for future behavior. That means you are more likely to repeat the same pattern the next time this situation or feeling comes up. The more you repeat it, the more natural it becomes, until it is what we call a habit. Once it becomes part of your behavior, it seems unnatural to act differently in the same situation. That is why we feel so comfortable eating unhealthy foods, even though we know they are not good for us. We have become conditioned to "feel" a certain way when we eat them and when we try to change our eating behavior; it feels like we are going against our desires. Once you change the associations that you have connected to certain foods or situations, it is easy to change your behavior. Until you do, you are trying to use willpower to go against your natural feelings creating a constant struggle.

How Did We Get This Way? Let's Blame Our Parents.

Associations to food start at an early age and continue through life. When a baby cries, the parents don't know what is wrong because the baby can't talk. They usually look for two likely problems. If the diaper is clean, they assume the baby is hungry. They pick up the baby and comfort it and then they give it a bottle. It could be that the baby is tired or cold, or any number of things that would make her cry. When the baby is picked up and held, she feels warmth and love and feelings of pleasure. By combining that feeling with a bottle, the baby begins to associate those good feelings of love and security to food.

It continues as the child grows. The young child falls down, skins her knee and comes in crying, "Mommy, Daddy! I hurt myself!" The well-meaning parent responds with, "Oh honey, sit down and have some milk and cookies and you'll feel better". This creates an association – "When I feel pain, food will make me feel better".

The young child comes home from school with her report saying, "Mommy, Daddy, look! I got three A's on my report card!"

The proud parent responds, "Oh, honey, that's great! Let's all go to Dairy Queen!" Now the child has a new association - when she feels good, food will make it even better.

Let me ask you this. When you are planning a party or any type of event, what is the first thing you think of? Food! In our society, we plan all of our activities with food. When we want to celebrate at the office, the boss brings in donuts.

How about cake? What do you associate cake with? The most common place to have cake is at a celebration. How could you have a wedding or birthday or anniversary without cake? Imagine this: You are at a party having fun and feeling wonderful. While you are in that emotional state of celebration, you eat the cake and it creates an association of feeling good to eating cake. Next week you go to another celebration and again they have cake. You're feeling excited and happy as you eat the cake. The association grows stronger. That's why eating cake gives us so much pleasure. Sure, it tastes good, but that's not the main reason we enjoy it. It makes us feel good because it brings back those good feelings. The next time you see a cake, it will trigger those good feelings and you will have a desire to eat cake.

Later on, we will see how we can create other associations that don't have calories. For now, be aware that these associations are being created throughout your life. Now it is time to take control of those associations.

Tipping the Scale

Think of your actions as putting weight on a scale. Every time you repeat an action, it puts more weight on the scale for that action. After a few times, it becomes a habit and you don't even have to think about it. A habit is nothing more than a conditioned response. When you see the stimulus, you react automatically without even thinking. The more you repeat it, the stronger it becomes.

When you change your action the first time, it starts to give your mind a new direction. Think of it like putting weight on the other side of the scale. You put on a small weight, but the other side has so much more weight from the repetition of your old behavior. If you don't reinforce that new action, your old programming will take over and you will return to your old behavior. Please realize that for some people, it will take more time to balance the scale in the other direction. That doesn't mean that changes are not occurring.

Imagine you are going on a trip from Los Angeles to Washington, D.C. If you change your course by only one degree, you will end up in Baltimore, Maryland. Every day you are changing your direction a little more, which leads you to a new destination. You will probably notice that you will begin to feel differently and you will notice your awareness is leading you where you direct it. You may go back to your old behavior the first few times, but when you keep putting weight on the other side of the scale, it will eventually tip in the direction you choose.

I'm going to show you some techniques that will help you put more weight on that scale even faster and make changes quickly. Just realize that when you stick with it, the change you desire will come quickly and easily.

Breaking the Conditioned Response through Awareness

If you have ever seen a rat in a maze, you will notice something very interesting that is very human-like. The rat will go down a path until it realizes it is a dead end, and then it comes back. The interesting part is that it will often go back down the same path, even though it knows there is a dead end. The rat knows it will not get out this way, but it also know it is safe this way. Nothing bad will happen. It is amazing how many people will go down the same path or repeat the same behavior, even though they know it will not give them the results they want. So, why do they do it? Because it has become a conditioned response!

Someone once told me the definition of stupidity is trying the same thing over and over and expecting a different result. If you've tried diets over and over without long-term success, you're likely to have the same result again. So, how do we break out of this rut? If the rat goes down the same path and you shock him, he will think twice about going that way again. He may still go back because it is still familiar. If you shock him again, he will probably start looking for a new path. That old comfort zone has suddenly become very uncomfortable.

You can do the same thing by "shocking" your nervous system to break that conditioned response. When you find yourself reaching for that chocolate or those chips and you know you are not hungry, throw out your hand in front of you, imagine seeing a stop sign and say, "Stop! That's not like me!"

The first time you do this, your mind may respond with, "Of course it is like me. I've been doing that for years". It's like the rat being shocked for the first time. It feels uncomfortable, but you've been down this road before and you may go down it again. The second time you do it, the resistance becomes stronger. After a few times, you may find yourself agreeing because you're now ready to go down a new path. If you want to make it even stronger, tell yourself what you want to do in this situation. Once you know what you don't want, you need to give yourself the direction of what you do want. Add the new behavior that you want on the end of your sentence to feed your subconscious. For example, "Stop! That's not like me! I now eat healthy foods like fruits and vegetables".

Three Ways to Make Changes

Here are the three basic ways to change your behavior. The first is repetition. When you repeat the same behavior over and over, it becomes a conditioned response and you don't have to think about it anymore. If you start a new job, move to a new home or just drive a new way to work, it takes the repetition of about 30 days to become ingrained in us.

This can happen with our tastes as well. I often ask people if they have switched from whole milk to skim milk. The people that have will say that when drinking whole milk, skim milk tasted like water. Now that they drink skim milk, whole milk tastes like heavy cream. When you start eating healthy foods, it may not connect like your old sweet or greasy food. Once you get used to it, the unhealthy food will taste too sweet or too greasy.

The second way to change your behavior is through a significant emotional event. I mentioned before that people will often go through their lives overweight, wanting to change, but not able to break free. Then they have some emotional event. It may be a negative event like being embarrassed or ashamed, or it may be positive like falling in love. Suddenly their feelings change and they find the ability to make permanent changes. When this happens, it is not

41

the ability or desire that changes. It is the emotion that adds fuel to the fire. If we combine these two methods, we can speed up the process even faster. If you repeat something with strong emotional feelings, even if you only repeat it in your mind, every occurrence will add to the other in a multiplying effect.

The third way you can change your behavior is to change your internal representations and feelings. I mentioned how we attach feelings of pleasure to celebration foods like cake. If we attach a new feeling to that cake, the desire will change. If you create feelings of pleasure to eating healthy foods, you will change your behavior to eat more healthy foods. We'll see several ways to do this in later chapters.

Keys to Successful Change

There are three keys to successfully change your behavior. If you don't have all three, you will find it much harder to create this change.

The first key is desire. As Napoleon Hill states in his classic book "Think and Grow Rich", you must have a burning desire for what you truly want. Most people have a wish for what they want or complain about what they have. You hear them say things like, "I wish I could lose some weight", or "I'm so sick of being fat". As you already know, words like these will not give your mind the direction it needs to achieve your goal. You have to first have a clear idea of what you want. Then you must create that burning desire to achieve your goal. The more you want it, the more you will move toward it. Think about some of your accomplishments for a moment. I'm sure that there were some things in your past that you wanted so much that you decided you would not settle for anything less. For some, it was getting a certain job or career. For others, it was spending years to complete a degree program or other academic learning. Maybe it was your dream vacation. Everyone has something they wanted enough that they found a way to get it. That is the same attitude you need here. You must create that burning desire to be the person you have chosen to become. It doesn't matter what you have done in the past. It is never too late to become the person you were meant to be.

The second key is belief. As Henry Ford said, "If you think you can or if you think you can't, you are always right". One phrase that always stuck in my mind was by Dr. Denis Waitley, who said, "It's not what you are that holds you back, it's what you think you are not". That is such a powerful message that I want you to go back and reread it. Whenever you say, "I'm not smart enough" or "I'm not good enough" or "I don't have the willpower" or anything else that you say you don't have enough of to be successful, you are limiting what you will be.

Part of this comes from the number of times a person hears what they can't do in their life. When you hear it enough, it limits what you believe you are capable of. When you tell yourself what you can't do, it reinforces that thought and you become trapped by your own beliefs. It is time to think like a child. If you ask a child what they want to be when they grow up, they have no limits. The ones that never learn to have limits as adults are the ones that change the world. In a few minutes, you will get a chance to identify your limiting beliefs. In a later chapter, you will learn how to collapse those beliefs and go beyond your old limits.

The third key is expectancy. There are many people who know what they are capable of, but never live up to it. It's not what you *can do* that creates a change; it's what you *will do* that makes it happen. When I was a corporate manager, I learned that most people will live up or down to your expectations. The same thing is true of each of us - we usually get just what we expect. If you expect to fail, you will find a way to fail. If you expect to succeed, you will find a way to succeed. Expect the best from yourself and your life. Once you do, doors will open like magic.

Belief: The Birth of Success (or Failure)

A belief is any guiding principle that provides a sense of certainty about meaning and direction in life. Here are six general reference sources that determine most beliefs:

Environment. Many of your beliefs were formed, or rather inherited, from your environment and the people around you. A good example of this is religion. Over seventy percent of adults who practice religious beliefs belong to the same religious organization they did as a child. I'm not saying there is anything wrong with this; I'm just saying that for most people it is not a conscious choice. Very few people gather information from all the available religions and make a decision on their religious preference. Most Catholics remain Catholics, most Protestants remain Protestants, most Hindus remain Hindus, etc.

How many of your beliefs are results of your environment rather than conscious thinking? If you have some limiting beliefs about yourself, where did they come from? Are they really yours or did someone else give them to you? Many of your beliefs came from your parents, your culture, your friends and even the other kids on the playground when you were little.

Past Events. Some of our beliefs come from the events in our lives that we have seen, heard about or experienced. For hundreds of years, no one believed a human being could run a mile in four minutes. After Roger Banister finally broke that barrier, hundreds of others did the same. It wasn't a physical barrier; it was a limiting belief.

Past Results. If you were successful at something in the past, you now have the belief that you can do it again. If you tried something in the past and it didn't work, you may have told yourself that you weren't capable of being successful at it. That may have been true then, but now you may have more knowledge or experience that will allow you to be successful. The past does not create the future unless you let it.

Knowledge. Knowledge is power. The more you know about something, the better your decisions can be. If you want to be good at anything, you have to study it.

Self Talk. We all talk to ourselves, whether we know it or not. Most of what we say to ourselves is negative. Have you ever caught yourself saying, "I can't believe I did something so stupid"?

On the other hand, have you ever given yourself a compliment? Try it right now. Tell yourself how good you are at something. When you do something well, tell yourself out loud how well you did it. I know it sounds silly, but it works. Most people spend time thinking about their faults and they forget about their good points.

Imagination of Future Events. Your subconscious mind cannot tell the difference between a real and a vividly imagined event. Since most of your actions are conditioned responses, you can create new responses for any situation. You don't have to be a slave to your past.

Identifying Your Limiting Beliefs

We all have beliefs about ourselves and our lives that are limiting what we can and will be. They may be beliefs about what we think we are capable of or even what we deserve. What beliefs do you have about yourself, your body and your ability to change?

Some common beliefs are:

"I'll never be able to lose weight."

"I can't stop eating sweets."

"I can't control myself".

"I don't believe I can change."

"No one in my family is thin. It must be in my genes."

What have you said to yourself in the past, even if you didn't think it was true? An easy way to find out is to say, "I'm heavy because _____."

Whatever follows the "because" is your belief.

You may be tempted to just say, "I'm heavy because I eat too much". Be sure to follow that up by asking yourself why you eat too much. What is the need you believe you have that you are filling with food? How do you think that is helping you?

Write down as many of your limiting beliefs as you can think of right now. Be sure to do this because we will use them in a later exercise.

1. _____

2. _____

3. _____

4. _____

5. _____

6. _____

7. _____

8. _____

9. _____

10. _____

Identifying Your Trigger Feelings

I always start working with individuals by asking, "When do you tend to overeat?" I ask them to finish this sentence:

"I eat when _____.

Then I hear answers like, "I eat when I'm bored, I eat when I'm lonely, I eat when I'm depressed", and a whole list of other reasons. The reason diets don't work is because they do not address these core issues or feelings that trigger the desire to eat. Write down all of your reasons for eating and we will use them in a later exercise.

I eat when:

_____

_____

_____

_____

_____

_____

_____

_____

It is never too late to become the person you were meant to be.

For a wrap-up of Chapter 2 go to
http://www.emotionaldiet.com/review.html.

Chapter Three

Create New Conditioned Responses

"Let's not forget that the little emotions are the great captains of our lives and we obey them without realizing it". ~Vincent Van Gogh -

S uccess or failure is based on what we believe our ability to be. This is not always constant. We start with what we believe our potential to be. Based on that belief, we take the action of which we think we are capable. Those actions create results. If the results are better than we expected, our belief about our potential goes up. If the results are less than expected, our beliefs of our capabilities may go down, thus our potential goes down. If we get what we expected (which is usually the case) it reinforces the current belief.

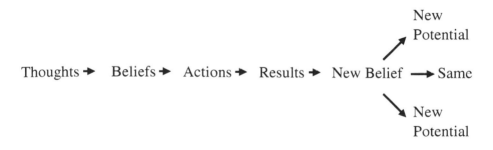

The easiest way to change your capabilities is to change your beliefs.

Key Beliefs of Successful People

It is important to remind ourselves that no matter how much we believe in an idea or concept, we should be open to other possibilities and new ideas. Here are some key beliefs that can be found again and again in successful people:

There are no failures. There are only results. We often tend to feel that if we don't reach our goal, we have failed. The only real failure is to not even try. As long as you do something, you will create a result. If it is not the result you wanted, try something else. Success is not just reaching your goal; it's becoming the person you want to be in the process.

Everything happens for a reason and it creates opportunities. I don't believe that things happen accidentally. The universe creates opportunities and opens doors for us. It is up to us to go through the door. Look for what you want with true expectations and you will find it.

Whatever happens, I take responsibility for my life. As I mentioned before, when we blame someone or something else for our situation, we become powerless to change. We are all living the life we choose. If you want your life to change, the choice must come from you.

I do not need to understand something to be able to use it. Some of the techniques you will learn may seem odd or too simple or even child-like. It is easy to dismiss something that you don't fully understand. You don't have to understand electricity to turn on the lights. You only need to know that when you flip the switch the lights do come on.

There is no lasting success until I commit to it. Wishing for something rarely creates success. When you commit to making something happen, it usually does. Promise yourself that you will commit to using these techniques for the next 30 days and you will see amazing changes.

Your Self Concept

This is the key to making positive changes in your life. You must be able to feel deserving, worthy, and capable of achieving your desired outcome. The negative self-talk you give yourself based on past results can tear down your self-esteem and limit your potential for change. Only by building your self-esteem and self worth can these issues be overcome and your personal power taken back.

One of my favorite business books is "The One Minute Manager". The simple concept is "catch people doing things right". How often have you caught yourself making a mistake and saying, "I can't believe how stupid I am". It is a common practice that most of us do. Now, how often do you catch yourself doing things right? Start telling yourself, "Wow, I really handled that situation well" or "I am really good at _____ (driving, shopping, listening, cooking, my job, helping others, etc.).

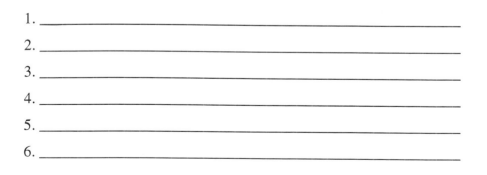

Make it a habit to catch yourself doing things right.
Value Yourself

Most people compare their worst traits to others best traits. We all have skills that we are good at. Most of us have been taught not to brag about ourselves. Because of that, we focus on our perceived "flaws" and ignore our skills. Now is the time to value yourself for your abilities and skills.

Write down 10 things that you like about yourself. This is no time to be modest. You have so many good qualities that it will be hard to stop at 10. If you have trouble with this (which most people do) ask yourself what your best friend would say about you. Are you a good friend, a good mother / father / sister / brother / daughter / son, a good worker, kind to animals, etc?

1. _____

2. _____

3. _____

4. _____

5. _____

6. _____

7. _____

8. _____

9. _____

10. _____

Your Special Place – A Metaphor for Your Life

Take a nice deep breath and close your eyes for a moment as you allow your body and mind to relax. Take another deep breath, and as you exhale, allow all of the tension to leave your body. Imagine now, that you are at the top of a beautiful stairway leading down to a special room. Notice the hand carved railing and the plush carpet runner that is your favorite color. As you begin to step down the stairs, you feel a wonderful sense of connection here. Your mind lets go of all other thoughts as you focus on the stairs. With every step, you become more relaxed and comfortable. 10...9...8...7...6...5...4...3...2...1.

When you get to the bottom of the stairs, you find yourself in a beautiful room that seems to have been put there just for you. In the middle of the room is a desk with a very comfortable looking chair. On top of the desk is a name plate with your name on it. As you sit down at the desk, you are surprised to find a large leather-bound book with your name in gold letters. You open the book and the first page comes to life with the scene of a beautiful baby being born. You somehow recognize the parents and realize that the baby is you. That's when it hits you; this is the book of your life.

As you turn the pages, you see images of your childhood – the places you played, the children you played with, it all comes rushing back. You turn more pages and see images of you as an older child. There is the school you attended and your teachers. You remember yourself going to classes and learning. You notice all of your friends and classmates.

As you continue to turn the pages, you find yourself back in high school. You see yourself at the places you went to, perhaps on dates or with friends.

You remember all of the happy times, and maybe even some that were not so happy. But mostly, you remember the people. You remember your friends, your family, all of the people that have been a part of your life.

As you turn more pages, you see yourself growing up. Perhaps it was at one of your first jobs. Maybe it was when you fell in love. There was so much to experience as you were growing up. Allow yourself to go back now and remember the people and places back then.

You begin to turn more pages now. You see yourself as a young adult. Think of all of the people that came into your life. Perhaps you remember some new friends and family members as your life changes in so many ways. So many people have been a part of your life in so many ways.

As you turn the pages faster, you begin to wonder – what would you find if you looked at the future? Could you see what will happen to you? You finally get to today and the page is only partially filled in. You look at tomorrow and it is blank. That is when you realize that the future is not yet written. The decisions you make today will determine what happens tomorrow. You suddenly get this feeling of having more power over your life than ever before. You realize that you control your own destiny.

As you think about what you might create in your future, your mind wanders back to all of the people that have been a part of your life, so far. There are so many people that have influenced you in so many ways. Now you begin to think of one person in particular that you care for, very much. It may be someone from your past or from your present. It may even be someone who is no longer a part of your life. As you think of this person, you begin to get the feeling that they are nearby. You look across the room and notice a glass door. There seems to be a faint image behind the door of the person you are thinking of, watching you with loving eyes. You smile to yourself, feeling so good about this person that cares so much for you.

You realize that in this special place, you have magical powers. You allow your spirit to drift out of your body, completely unnoticed by the person who is watching you. You float across the room and right through the wall, coming out next to this person. You look back through the window and see yourself as they see you. You see the beautiful, wonderful, caring person that you are. You have never seen yourself like this and you love what you see.

You look at the face of the person next to you and you begin to wonder what they are feeling. You gently and tenderly float into their body and suddenly feel all of their thoughts and feelings. You see yourself through their eyes, the eyes of love, and you feel all the love they have for you. You notice their thoughts and memories about you and all of the other people that care for you. You remember all of the people that you have helped and somehow played a part in their lives. There are so many people that you have touched in your life. You begin to realize how important your life has been to so many people. It feels so good to know that your life has had so much meaning.

Then you think of all of the people you will touch in the future. There is so much more waiting for you. You realize that the greatest gift you can give to all of the people that care about you is a happier, healthier you. Now, you decide that you will take better care of your body and enjoy the experience of being alive.

As you float out of this person, you take with you all of the love you feel. You know that you cannot love others fully and completely until you love yourself and you promise to love yourself as much as others love you from now on.

You float back into your body, feeling so good about yourself and your life. You write down in your book all that you have learned. Then, you close your book and leave, knowing that you will return to learn more in the future.

Your actions are not you

What are some behaviors in regard to health and eating that you have and you know you should change but haven't changed? How does that make you feel? Write down these behaviors followed by one word that best describes how you feel about each one.

Behavior   Feeling

_____   _____

_____   _____

_____   _____

_____   _____

_____   _____

Now ask yourself this question - "Do these behaviors make me a bad person?"

Of course, the answer is "NO". Your actions are not you. Just because you may have made some unhealthy choices in the past, it does not make you a bad person. You are simply a good person who has some behavior you want to change. Instead of beating yourself up for this behavior, ask yourself what you can learn from this and how you can act differently next time. Go back and cross out the words you used to describe your feelings now.

Forgiveness is the key; Learning is the reward

Why verses How - Asking Better Questions

Imagine that you have been eating healthy all day. Suddenly something happens to raise your anxiety level. Maybe you worry about something at work or you have a deadline to meet. You look over on your coworker's desk and you see a big bowl of candy. Your anxiety goes higher, so you reach for a handful of candy. The candy momentarily gives you pleasure, but then you think about how you just blew your diet. Then you get angry for giving into temptation.

55

What do you ask yourself at this point? That's right. You ask, "Why did I do that?" That is the worst thing you can do. There is a part of your mind that has a need to rationalize everything you do.

When you ask, "Why did I do that?" your mind starts searching for an answer. It will usually come up with answers like "Because you have no willpower, because you can't control yourself, because you're weak, because you're a loser", and the list goes on and on.

When your mind comes up with these answers, do they empower you? No! They just reinforce the false belief that you can't change. Every time you ask yourself questions like that, you reinforce those same beliefs that trap you in the same behavior.

So, what can you do? The first step is to stop beating yourself up. Eating excess food does not make you a bad person. You're a good person with behavior that you would like to change.

Next, ask yourself empowering questions. These usually start with "How". For example, "How can I do that differently next time?" The first thing that happens with a question like this is that it creates a presupposition that you can do it differently. That makes you feel more resourceful. Since your mind has a need to find an answer, it searches until you find a way to do things differently next time. You may decide that when you feel stressed, instead of eating candy, you'll go for a walk or take 3 deep breaths or hum a song that makes you feel happy.

You have the resources to find the answer. When you talk about negative behavior, always ask empowering questions. "Why" questions will find problems and "How" questions will find answers. You can even set yourself up for success by asking yourself, "How can I do this differently next time and enjoy it even more than food?"

The empowering thought is that you will find a different way and you will enjoy it more than food. With a solution like that, why would you turn to food? Once you decide on a new behavior, you have to program yourself for the future. Just imagine that you are in the same situation again and imagine yourself using your new behavior. Make it as real as possible. Then congratulate yourself for your new behavior and allow yourself to feel really proud.

New Behavior Exercise

Think back to a previous time you ate too much food or unhealthy food. Where were you? What emotions were you feeling? Were you alone or with someone?

Now, write down the new behavior you will use the next time you are in this situation. It is important to write it because it clarifies your thoughts and gives them life. There is amazing power in writing down what you want.

_____

_____

_____

_____

_____

_____

Now, imagine that you are in the same situation again and notice how you use your new behavior so easily and powerfully. Live the experience in your mind the way you wrote it down. Make the experience as real as possible. You are now programming yourself for a new conditioned response and a new behavior.

Secondary Gain

When you continue a certain behavior, it is because you gain something from your actions. What do you get by holding on to this behavior? What are the benefits of not changing? It may be the pleasure of eating. It may be some emotional need that is being fulfilled. For some people, food is a companion or certain foods are connected to feelings. Others may get a feeling of security from eating because it is something they can control.

One person I worked with realized that she had gained weight after the painful break-up of what seemed to be a wonderful relationship. As she thought back to that time, she remembered how she had turned to food to fill a void in her life. When we searched deeper, we found that she had a subconscious fear of another painful break-up. Holding on the excess weight kept her from feeling attractive and kept her from getting into another relationship where she could get hurt again. When she let go of the pain from the memory and let go of her limiting beliefs, she was able to let go of the excess weight easily and open her life to a new relationship.

Think of what you gain by eating too much or eating unhealthy foods. Allow yourself to search your feelings. Write down as many ideas as you can. We will use these for a later exercise.

Eating gives me:

1. _____

2. _____

3. _____

4. _____

5. _____

Creating Emotional Leverage for Change

As I have said many times, we are not driven by logic, we are driven by emotion. If you want to create a change, you need to create emotional leverage that drives you to create that change. Since you have attached positive emotions to eating, those emotions have been taking you down the path that satisfies those emotions. This exercise will help you change the emotional ties to eating that have held you captive.

What has it cost you in your life?

Write down 5 ways that having this extra weight has cost you in your life so far. What have you missed in your life that you might have had? How do you think this has held you back in your personal and professional life? How does that make you feel? Really engage your emotions and feelings.

1. _____
2. _____
3. _____
4. _____
5. _____

What will it cost you if you don't change?

Write down 5 ways that it will cost you in the future if you don't change. Don't just say, "I will be heavy". Write down what it will cost you physically, emotionally, in your social life, in your self-image. Be specific and include your feelings.

1. _____
2. _____
3. _____
4. _____
5. _____

What will you gain when you do change?

Write down 10 ways that your life will improve when you do change. Really think about these and how it will make your life better. Be specific and include your feelings. As you do, allow yourself to imagine that these changes have already happened, and see how good that makes you feel.

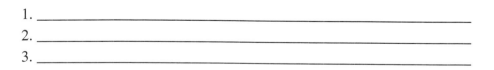

1. _____
2. _____
3. _____

4. _____

5. _____

6. _____

7. _____

8. _____

9. _____

10. _____

Keep all of these thoughts and images in the forefront of your mind. As I said before, one reason it is hard to stick to a healthy diet is because of the proximity of the object you desire. If you see your favorite unhealthy food in front of you, it is immediate. The trim, healthy body is somewhere in the future. It is so easy to choose whatever is closest.

If you could walk through that door on your left and have your favorite food, or walk through that door on the right and be trim and healthy *right now*, you would choose the trim healthy body. Remember that every day your goal is to peel off one or two strips of bacon from your body. Not in the future, but today. When you look at that food, see the bacon sitting on the plate with it. If you eat the unhealthy food (or overeat any food), imagine that you are putting a strip of fat bacon on your body. When you choose to pass up that food, you are peeling a strip of fat bacon off your body.

The Road to the Future – a Metaphor for Change

Take a nice deep breath and close your eyes for a moment as you allow your body and mind to relax. Take another deep breath, and as you exhale, allow all of the tension to leave your body. Imagine now, that you are at the top of a beautiful stairway leading down to your special room. Notice the hand carved railing and the plush carpet runner that is your favorite color. As you begin to step down the stairs, you feel a wonderful sense of connection here. Your mind lets go of all other thoughts as you focus on the stairs. With every step, you become more relaxed and comfortable. 10…9…8…7…6…5…4…3…2…1.

When you get to the bottom of the stairs, you find yourself back in the beautiful room that was put here just for you. In the middle of the room is the desk with that very comfortable chair. You sit down at the desk, open the book of your life and turn to today. As you look at the partially filled page, you wonder what the future will bring. You stare at the blank pages of tomorrow and the next day. As you sit there deep in thought, your eyes focus on a door across the room with the word "Future" written on it. You wonder what you might find on the other side of that door. You walk across the room, passing through the door to the future, curious about what you will find there.

As you walk through the doorway, you come to a path with a fork that goes in two directions. The path on the left takes you back down the road you have been on for so many years. The old path is easy because it goes downhill, which is how you feel your life has been going. The path to the right leads to the new path you have chosen, a life of health and happiness. The new path takes more effort because you climb to new heights becoming more than you were before. It is much like climbing a mountain. The higher you climb, the better the view. And now, you really want to see the world as a trim and healthy person.

You decide to venture back down the old path to see what your life would be like if you return to your old behavior. With every step, you go a year into the future. After the first step, you notice a feeling of remorse because you have spent one more year wishing your life was different but nothing has changed. You continue, two, three, four, five years into the future. You stop to look around. You notice that it has become harder to walk and you are breathing heavily. Your weight has gone up and you can feel the difference. You feel tired and lethargic, with little energy.

You head down the path again. Six, seven, eight, nine, ten years into the future. You can feel the toll that 10 more years of poor food and lack of exercise has taken on your body. Your blood pressure is higher and you have signs of diabetes and heart disease. You look back down the path of ten more years of disappointments, always wishing you would have changed your life but never doing it. The path is littered with junk food wrappers, shattered dreams and broken promises. This isn't the life you wanted, but it is the life you have chosen. You feel an overwhelming feeling of disappointment, knowing it could have been different and wishing you could go back and do it over.

As you look back down the path, you realize that you still have a choice. You start back down the path.....nine, eight, seven, six, five, four, three, two, one, and you find yourself back at the fork in the path.

You look down the path to the right – the path you have already started down. With every step you go one year into the future – a future of healthy living and happiness. After the first step, you feel energized and excited. You remember feeling better and happier the first day. You are now living the life of your dreams. Two, three, four, five more years of healthy food and exercise. You notice how much more energy you have. You feel lighter and calmer. A feeling of confidence comes over you. You can't wait to continue.

Six, seven, eight, nine, ten years of healthy living. You look in the mirror and see how trim and healthy you have become. People around you tell you how fantastic you look. Your life has become exactly the way you always wanted. Your energy is sky high and you have accomplished so much. You have never felt so alive.

As you look back down the path, you see so many other changes that have taken place in your life. Changing your behavior and associations was only the beginning. You have applied the same principles to other areas of your life and your life has improved in so many ways. A sense of pride and contentment comes over you as you realize that all of the changes have come from you.

As you think about how wonderful the past ten years have been, you realize that you get to go back and live it all over again. There are so many experiences that you will enjoy. Your life is going to be magical. The excitement comes over you as you travel back down the path, with each step taking you a year back in time until you come to the doorway of today.

You sit back down at your desk and write in your book what you have learned. You have seen your future and you love what you have seen. You write down your new feelings, your new behavior and everything you have created in your new life. You close your book now, knowing that you will come back and visit this special place again.

For a wrap-up of Chapter 3 go to
http://www.emotionaldiet.com/review.html.

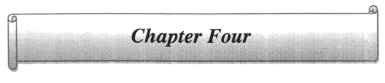

Chapter Four

Creating Change Now

"When we are no longer able to change a situation, we are challenged to change ourselves". ~Victor Frankl-

You already know that the key to directing your thoughts is having a clear picture of the results you want. If you created your blueprint for success and you focus on it every morning, your thoughts, feelings and actions will come in line with your desired outcome. Now we are going to focus on how you can change your thoughts and feelings to create new actions or new behavior.

Here is the basic model of cognitive behavior:

Thoughts = Feelings = Action = Results

Almost everything people do is a conditioned response, sometimes referred to as a habit. What we often call habits, especially when we talk about eating, are not really simple habits. For example, if you get up every morning and put on your right shoe first and then your left shoe, that is a habit. You don't think about it, you just do it the same way every time because it is a repeated behavior.

When you eat too much or eat the wrong kind of food, it is a response to the stimulus and how you have become conditioned to feel about that particular food. This is much like Ivan Pavlov demonstrated with dogs. He fed them and rang a bell. After repeating this several times, they had associated the bell to food and began to salivate at the sound of the bell.

People do the same thing with their food. We create associations to feelings and when we see the food, we experience emotion like pleasure, and act just like the dogs. The way to create change is to alter the way we feel about the stimulus, or the feelings connected to the food.

There are many ways that you can create change in your thinking and your behavior. Now I am going to introduce several methods for changing your associations. All of these have been proven to work for the majority of people. If you use any one of these repeatedly, with feeling, you will be able to create the change you desire. I have never been a believer of the "one size fits all" approach. Try each of these and find out which ones work best for you. If you combine several of them together, you will create change even faster.

Change Your Focus

Whenever we evaluate something, it is usually based on what we will gain and what we will lose. With food, we look at it and think, "What will I gain if I eat this and what will I lose if I don't?" Imagine someone brings a box of donuts into your work place or someplace where you gather. You look at the donuts and think, "If I eat one, I'll have the pleasure of the taste. If I don't have one now, there may not be any later". You've just told yourself that you will gain something if you eat a donut and you will lose something if you don't eat one. With a Win/Lose mind set like this, you are probably going to eat the food every time. It becomes the scarcity mentality.

Now, reverse the options. Ask yourself, "What will I gain if you pass up the food and what will I lose if I eat it"? Imagine feeling heavy, sluggish and bloated if you eat the food. Then imagine feeling healthy, energized and full of vitality when you pass up the unhealthy food. Notice how good it feels to be in control instead of being controlled by food. Connect unpleasant feelings to eating the excess food, and connect good feelings to passing up the food.

Think of the Ingredients

Would you sit down with a big bowl of white flour and a spoon, and just eat it? That probably does not sound very appealing. How about sitting down to a big bowl of white processed sugar? For some people, that may sound better but still not very appealing. It also creates thoughts of rotting your teeth out. Let's try one more. Would you sit down with a big can of Crisco shortening and a spoon and start eating? That sounds really repulsive, doesn't it?

Let me ask you this – what if we mixed them all together and called them donuts? Aha – now you are getting a different picture, aren't you? So the real question is, if you would not eat each of these ingredients alone, does it make sense to eat them together? I explained this to one client I worked with who loved donuts. She has not eaten another donut since then because now when she sees a donut, she mentally imagines that donut as a ring of solid Crisco. Her old association of pleasure has now been replaced with the thought of how it would taste and feel to have solid Crisco in her mouth.

Think of some unhealthy foods that you have eaten to excess in the past. What are some ingredients that come to mind that you would not eat alone? Now, imagine that this food is filled with that ingredient (which it really is). Imagine how it would feel and taste to have a mouth full of that single ingredient. If you thought of shortening, imagine how it would taste and feel to have a mouthful of Crisco. It's not very appealing, is it? Repeat this three or four more times and you will probably find that this food is no longer as attractive as it was. You may even notice that it actually seems unattractive and you have lost some or all of your desire for it.

Bring the Future to the Present

Why is it so hard to pass up food when you know that you want to be trim and healthy? The reason is because you are torn between two desires. Part of you wants to be trim and healthy while part of you wants to eat that food that has given you pleasure in the past. The one that draws you the most is not necessarily the one that you feel is most important. Remember, we are not driven by logic, we are driven by emotion. In this case, the emotion you are feeling is desire. The desire that will usually win is the one that is the closest. Right now, the chocolate is sitting right in front of you, while your goal of being at a certain weight or size seems months in the future. That makes it so easy to say, "I'll start my diet tomorrow". Does that sound familiar?

Now, let's change the scenario. Remember the two doors right in front of you? The door on the left leads to the food you desire. The door on the right leads to the body you desire. The door you go through will give you what you desire right now. You can either have the food you desire or the body you desire just by going through one of these doors. Which one will you choose? I know you've heard this before. Do this every time you feel tempted until it becomes automatic.

At the end of the last chapter, you went on an imaginary journey into the future that took you to a choice of two paths. The path on the left leads to overeating, obesity and poor health. The path on the right leads to great health, vitality and a trim, healthy body.

Every day you take a step down one of these paths. The future is right now. Every time you look at food (especially the unhealthy food), bring a picture into your mind. On the left side, see the future of you looking heavy and feeling tired and sluggish. On the right, see the other you, looking trim and healthy, feeling so incredibly alive.

As you imagine both futures side by side, realize that your choice right now will take you one step into one of these futures. Keep both of them in front of you every time you think about food and exercise. Both of these futures are here right now. What you do today will affect you today. By seeing and feeling the pain of being heavy and at the same time, seeing and feeling the pleasure of looking and feeling great, you will bring the desire to be trim and healthy into the present moment. The brighter and closer you make it, the more it will affect you. Remember, the desire that is the closest is usually the most appealing.

Self-Talk - Your Words Drive Your Feelings

Do you talk to yourself? That's OK, we all do that. Unfortunately, most of what we say to ourselves is negative. Do you ever catch yourself saying things like, "That was really stupid", or "I can't believe I did that!" When you say something like that, your subconscious hears every word. After awhile you begin to believe what you have told yourself whether it is true or not. When you tell yourself, "I always eat too much", do you know what you are programming yourself to do? That's right! You're programming yourself to eat too much. Whatever behavior or feeling you tell yourself you have, you will create.

Now, let's look at the other side. Do you ever tell yourself how good you are? Try it right now. Think of something you have done well today. It may be as simple as driving a car or cleaning your home. Maybe you are a good parent or a good friend. Think back to the list of things you like about yourself. Now tell yourself how good you are at something or how proud you are of something you've done.

The first time you do this, it will probably seem strange. The more you do it, the better it will feel. You need to love and appreciate yourself. Catch yourself doing things right. Stop telling yourself what you are doing wrong and start telling yourself what you are doing right. Either way, you are reinforcing your behavior. Wouldn't it be better to reinforce the behavior you want?

Your Words Have Power

The words we use are so powerful and they influence how we live our lives. Research shows that our choice of words can manifest into our realities. When you talk, you create mental images with feelings attached. Most people are not even aware of the internal feelings that they are projecting when they talk. How many times have you ever said "something is killing me" or someone is a "pain in the neck" or some other part of the body. Imagine what kind of affect this has had on your body.

Notice the words you use talking to others. Notice the words in your head. What is the meaning of the words you use? For example:

"This job is killing me!"

"I am dead tired!"

Now consider what kinds of affects you could have on your body if you now begin to use words that promote health and healing. "I feel fantastic," is just one example of the idiomatic expressions you may begin to use. That is my favorite phrase.

Have you ever noticed how people always ask, "How are you doing?" And then you answer with something like, "Not bad for a Monday", or "I'm getting by". Do you really want a life that is "just getting by"? If you want a fantastic life, answer that question by saying, "I am FANTASTIC!" You will notice a great deal of difference in how you feel by carefully choosing the specific word you use to convey a meaning.

Notice the difference in the feeling you get from the following words:

Enraged and Angry vs. Upset, Annoyed or Peeved

Depressed, Down and Sad vs. Blue or Occupied

Exhausted, Worn out, Pooped vs. Tired or Fatigued

Also notice the difference of the positive words you use:

Happy vs. Elated, Excited, Ecstatic

Good vs. Great, Fantastic, Incredible

Okay vs. Outstanding, Extraordinary, Exceptional

Consider the following statement that many people use when they are hungry – "I am famished!" Now, compare that to someone saying, "I am getting a bit hungry". Both describe the same feeling – a desire for food. However, they create a different feeling and a different level of desire for the food. Which one is more likely to create a behavior that would drive you to overeat? You may be thinking, "What if I am really hungry? What if I am famished?" Think of the idea of a famine and ask if you have ever really suffered like that. Even if you are really hungry, you will tend to feel less like overeating if you mildly say that you are just a bit hungry. You create the feeling you want by the words you use.

Your phrases can also help determine your level of desire when you describe food. Have you ever heard someone say, "That dessert is to die for"? Would you get a different level of desire if the same person said, "That dessert is good"?

The words you say to yourself can also have a lot of power. Let me show you what I mean.

Right now, say this out loud with feeling – *"I hate being fat!"* How did it feel? For most people, it's not very good. Hate is a very powerful emotion, and just using the word can bring feelings that are associated with it. When you say, "I hate being fat", where are you directing those feelings? If you are like most people, you are directing them toward yourself.

Now, say this out loud with feeling - *"I love being trim and healthy!"* Did you feel the difference? Love is also a very powerful emotion. When you say this, you are associating this powerful emotion with the idea of being trim and healthy. You will never become trim and healthy with a mindset that says "I hate being fat". When you focus on being fat, you create more of what you focus on. Your self-talk can direct your focus.

Here is an easy way to keep focused in the right direction. Several times throughout the day, just say out loud (or to yourself if you are in a crowd), "I love being trim and healthy". When you say it, bring back the image of yourself as the person you intend to be. The more you repeat this exercise, the more it directs your subconscious mind to create the behavior that matches your image. By saying this with feeling, as you imagine yourself as the person you want to be, you engage multiple senses which will accelerate the changes.

Here is an exercise you can use in the morning when you first get up or when you go to bed at night. Go into the bathroom, look at yourself in the mirror and tell yourself how much you love yourself. Then, smile and tell yourself why you are proud of yourself. Get used to talking to yourself every day. You deserve to feel good about yourself, and you have so much to be proud of.

There are many words in the English language with emotional value. Why not begin to use the words that make you feel more ecstatic, more phenomenal, and more fantastic, so that you can live an exceptional life?

Here are a couple more phrases you might want to use:

> Nothing tastes as good as being trim and healthy.

> Nothing tastes as good as trim and healthy feels.

> I love feeling good about myself and my body.

> I love being trim and healthy.

Make your own signs that inspire you. Put them around your house or your work place. Put a screen saver on your computer. Put them everywhere you want to feel better.

Interrupt Your Automatic Conditioned Responses

I mentioned this earlier and it is worth repeating because it is very effective. Remember what happens if you put a rat in a maze with several dead ends? It will go down the first one until it finds a dead end. Then it will come back. What is interesting is that it will usually turn around and go back down the same path, even though there is no escape. The reason is because the rat knows how to get there and back and the path is familiar. The more it travels down that path, the more likely it is to repeat this pattern. After a few times down that path, the pattern becomes part of the rat's behavior. If you shock the rat while it goes down that path, it will decide that this is not a good way to go anymore and will look for another way.

People often fall into self-perpetuating patterns of negative or destructive behavior. Interrupting that behavior pattern with a totally unexpected action can have lasting effects by erasing that pattern from that person's behavior while replacing it with a new, empowering pattern.

Recently, I worked with a woman who was suffering from panic attacks. I asked her to tell me, in detail about one of her recent attacks and relive the experience as much as possible. As she started describing the experience, she became visibility uncomfortable. Her palms started to sweat, her legs started to shake and her voice became very shaky. At that point, I reached over and squeezed her nose as I said, "Honk!"

She stopped instantly and looked back at me with a surprised look on her face. "I'm sorry", I said. "Sometimes I just get this uncontrollable urge to honk someone's nose. It's just so much fun that I can't help myself". What I had done was interrupted her conditioned response that caused her to panic when she remembered that experience. "Go ahead and finish your story", I said. "What?" she answered. "You were telling me about your experience", I replied. "Please go on".

It took her a minute to get back to the same point in the experience, but this time she was not as intense. As her intensity started to climb again, I reached over and honked her nose again. "What are you doing?" she asked with a smile. "I guess I just lost control again", I answered. "You just have such a great nose for honking".

That brought a smile from her as she said, "You are making it hard for me to concentrate on my experience". "OK", I answered, "I'll try to control myself". At this point she was no longer showing the signs of panic and she was having a hard time connecting with the feelings of the experience. I asked her to continue and I could tell her response to the memory was changing. As she got back into the story, I playfully pretended like I was going to honk her nose again and she broke out laughing. I explained how the idea of honking her nose was creating a feeling of fun, which didn't match the feeling of panic from the experience. She decided that from now on, whenever she started to feel signs of panic she would just honk her nose and feel playful.

You can do the same thing if you have an urge to eat when you are not hungry. Realize that you are responding to the emotional condition that you are feeling at the time. The first step is to interrupt the conditioned response.

When you notice you are acting out of a habit (caught in the maze), stop and say to yourself, "STOP! That's not like me". You might even hold your hand up like a police officer would do to stop a car. Imagine a street sign with a picture of food and a circle with a line through it for "No Overeating". You could also do something pleasant like humming or singing your favorite song or get up and dance. You can even honk your nose, if you like. Just do anything that snaps you out of that automatic urge to reach for food. The more you do this, the more effective it becomes. By saying a phrase like "That's not like me" or "I'm in control now", you will begin to reprogram yourself with your own words.

> When you notice you are acting out of a habit (caught in the maze), stop and say to yourself, "STOP! That's not like me".

Notice Your Feelings

One of the main reasons for overeating is because someone is feeling an emotional need. Almost everything we do is because we want to feel better. When you feel lonely, stressed or just a bit down, you know that certain foods will make you feel better. Unfortunately, that is just a temporary quick-fix.

So, what are feelings for and why do we have them? They really do have a purpose. Most people spend so much time trying to avoid or change their feelings that they never really stop to notice them and what their feelings are trying to tell them. Again, think of your feelings as you would think of the gauges on your car. When your oil light comes on, it is telling you that something is wrong. Putting more gas in the car will not fix the problem. It may take your mind off the oil light momentarily, but you are not addressing the real need.

When you try to suppress your feelings by putting more food in your body, you are also not addressing the real need. You are only reinforcing the habit of trying to suppress the feeling, but the real problem is still there. Instead of ignoring your real feelings, ask yourself what you are feeling. Be honest with yourself. You might even try asking as though you are your own best friend trying to help yourself feel better.

When you identify the feeling, identify the cause of that feeling. If you are feeling lonely, what is causing you to feel lonely? If you are angry, what are you really angry about? If you are sad, what is the cause of your sadness? Once you identify the feeling, you can deal with that instead of using food to try to change the way you feel. In a later chapter, you will see how you can release the feelings that you are trying to tranquilize with food.

Write down the feelings you identify and any related causes that might have come up. If you are not sure where the feeling came from, just focus on the feeling and see if it comes up later.

Feeling	Cause
_____	_____
_____	_____
_____	_____
_____	_____
_____	_____
_____	_____
_____	_____

Tracking Your Eating Habits

Now it is time to identify the feelings and places that trigger your desire to eat. Just raising your awareness can start to change your feelings.

For some people it may be a certain time of the day. For others it may be a place they associate with food or eating. You may find that a particular emotion like frustration or loneliness will trigger a desire to eat. It may be that you just don't realize the times you have a little snack or the handful of French Fries that your child didn't finish.

One of the most effective ways of raising your awareness and creating change is to keep an eating diary. By tracking your eating, you avoid the mindless eating that can add on those extra pounds. One thing that a typical eating diary does not do is identify the feelings and emotions that trigger the desire to eat. If you have a desire to eat when you are not hungry, find out what emotional need you are filling with food.

You can download a printable copy of this eating record at
http://www.emotionaldiet.com/downloads.html.

For a wrap-up of Chapter 4 go to http://www.emotionaldiet.com/review.html.

Eating Record

Day _____

Time / Place   Emotion / Cause

_____   _____

_____   _____

_____   _____

_____   _____

_____   _____

_____   _____

_____   _____

_____   _____

_____   _____

_____   _____

Chapter Five

Making Changes with NLP

"If you don't like something change it; if you can't change it, change the way you think about it". ~Mary Engelbreit

Neuro-Linguistic Programming (NLP) is a behavioral technology, which allows you to change, adopt, or eliminate behaviors and allows you to choose your mental, emotional and physical states of well-being.

The neurological system (Neuro) controls how your body functions. Language (Linguistics) determines how you communicate with yourself and other people. Programming determines the kinds of models of the world we create. With NLP, you can change the way you feel about past and future experiences and the world around you. Some of the techniques you have already learned are variations of NLP techniques. Here are some specific techniques that will help you create even stronger changes.

Change Your Experience

The structure of how we experience life is based upon a human being's five senses, also known as modalities. They are: visual, auditory, kinesthetic, olfactory (smell), and gustatory (taste). Each of these modalities is composed of components called sub modalities. Examples would be color and brightness for visual and volume, tone and tempo for auditory. When you change your modalities and sub modalities, you change your view of your experience.

Right now, imagine your favorite food. Maybe it's a big juicy hamburger or pastry or chips. Imagine it in front of you, right now. Feel free to close your eyes if it makes the experience more real. As you imagine that food you like so well, notice how it appears in your mind's eye. Is it near or far away? Is it in color or black and white? Is it clear or fuzzy? Most people will say that it is near, in color and clearly focused. Now, bleed all the color out of the picture so that all you see is shades of gray, black and white. Make the image a bit fuzzy and out of focus. Now, move it farther away. Did it seem to lose some of its appeal?

Let's change it the other way. Bring it back even closer that it was before. Make it clear and colorful. Make the colors even brighter and more vivid. Imagine smelling the delicious aroma of this food you enjoy so much. Does it seem even more appealing now? For most people, the desire for this food goes way up. That is exactly what commercials do to you. The more often you see the same commercial, the more your desire goes up for that juicy burger or whatever you have in mind.

The way you use your mind to store your thoughts about a certain food will determine your desire for it. That means you can easily lose your desire for unhealthy foods and increase your desire for healthy foods. Let's do some more of that right now.

Think of a bag of those cheese curls that come in a plastic bag. These are the long, puffed snacks made of processed corn meal with orange cheese of some type covering them. You may or may not already be fond of these, but we'll use them for this exercise. You can repeat the process for any food you like. Imagine that you have a large bag of these cheese curls in front of you, right now. Imagine that you open the bag, look inside, and smell the aroma of the cheese curls. Now, imagine that you grab a handful and put one in your mouth right now and start to eat it. How does that experience appear in your mind right now? Of course, this can vary, depending on whether or not you enjoy these snacks. Most people will say the snacks seem very close, clear and bright orange. They feel crunchy to the touch and to chew, with the odor and taste of cheese. If you have ever tasted these, you can re-experience that easily.

Now, let's change the experience. Imagine that the corn curls are in front of you in a much smaller bag and a bit farther away. Let all of the color go from the bag and the snacks so that they are black and white, with shades of gray. You notice the list of ingredients and realize that they are mostly chemicals and processed by-products. You notice the bag is already opened, so they may be a bit stale. Imagine that you reach in the bag and feel that they are a bit damp and soggy, with no crispness at all. There is a moldy odor coming from the bag. You pull out a hand full of the limp, musty, gray snacks that now have a strong resemblance to large earthworms. As you bring one to your mouth, the odor becomes stronger. You put it in your mouth and notice the limp, sloppy texture and the moldy taste that matches the smell. Go ahead and spit it out. You don't want to eat these. They are not real food anyway. OK, how appealing are they right now? For most people, the appeal is gone and they have actually become unappealing.

Now let's do the reverse. Imagine you see a bowl of fresh, colorful fruit in front of you. There are oranges, apples, strawberries and other delicious, natural fruits in the bowl. You notice how bright red and fresh these strawberries look. They are nice and cool, with little drops of moisture on them. You reach down and pick one up, and it feels so cool and refreshing. You can smell that delicious aroma of sweet freshness; just the way nature had intended it to be. As you bring it up to your mouth, you think of how healthy berries are. You take a bite of the beautiful red, juicy strawberry and experience a splash of wonderful flavor in your mouth. As you swallow the tasty morsel, you can feel every cell in your body being energized and refreshed.

Now, which would you rather have at this moment? If you really allowed yourself to experience this, you let go of your desire for the unhealthy food and increased your desire for the healthy food. If you had a hard time really creating this experience, try having someone read this to you (or record it and play it back) as you close your eyes.

Does this mean that you will never eat corn curls again? Not necessarily, although you may think of them differently now. If you repeat this type of exercise several more times, you will notice a change. For some people, it only takes a couple of times. For others, it may take more repetitions because you have a stronger association to certain foods that you overeat. If you spend just a few minutes doing this every day, you will notice that your taste will change and you will shift your desire to healthy food.

There are many ways to make a food seem unappealing. In my seminars, I ask people to find their own ways to makes their favorite unhealthy food less appealing. The creative ideas are just amazing. Some people have made soda warm or flat. Some have made chocolate old with a white, chalky coating that you see when it has been around too long. Others have made the chocolate have a texture that is waxy and hard to swallow.

Some people have imagined the food being visited by other creatures, such as having a fly or ants crawl on the food. They have even mentioned noticing dirt or mold inside the cakes and donuts. One person even suggested seeing worms crawling on the food. That was a really interesting visual. The main thing is that it worked for her and many others in the seminar.

Another very effective way to change your associations is to engage the rest of your senses. Make the texture greasy or unnatural, make the aroma something that is unpleasant to you, such as rotting garbage, hear unpleasant sounds or hear someone saying, "Oh, no! No one would eat that!"

One of the best examples I can think of is when a woman tried to scam Wendy's hamburger chain by claiming that she had discovered a finger in her chili. It turned out to be a fraud, but it cost Wendy's millions of dollars because it planted that image in people's minds and they lost their desire for Wendy's chili and other food on their menu.

Right now, write down 5 foods that you have eaten in the past that you know are unhealthy. Then take each one and change it in your mind to make it less appealing. Change the color, smell, taste, texture; even make it old and moldy if you like. Do this at least twice for each food.

1. _____

2. _____

3. _____

4. _____

5. _____

Now write down five foods that are healthy. They don't have to be foods that you already enjoy. You can even take foods that you didn't enjoy in the past and make them appealing. Use the same process to change the color, closeness, freshness, anything that would make them more appealing to you. If they are foods that you don't care for, imagine them combined with foods you do like and notice how much you enjoy them now. Allow your body to feel energized and healthy from eating these foods. Do this twice for each food.

1. _____

2. _____

3. _____

4. _____

5. _____

Using Anchors

We have been talking about the associations that we create throughout life and the conditioned responses that we often attach to them. Another type of association is called an anchor. Anchor is an NLP term for what occurs when your mood changes in response to some trigger or stimulus.

Anchors are created when we are in a highly emotional state and we engage any of our senses. Many people can hear a certain song and it will take them back to a particular time and place that connects with a feeling. Whenever I smell the exhaust of a diesel truck, I have flashbacks to my days in the Army as a heavy truck driver.

Advertisers use this all the time. Let's say you're watching TV. You see a commercial for a certain food and you hear the voice of a famous celebrity but you never see their face. Then you hear some of your favorite music in the background. You feel good as you hear the music and then you see their product. The next time you see their product, those feelings come back and you have a desire to buy their product. That's an example of anchoring.

This did not happen by accident. You and your children have been educated by the snack food industry to respond in this way. They spend lots of money turning us into couch potatoes by setting up anchors such as these to get us to feel a desire for their products.

Here are some common pleasant anchors:

- The smell of freshly baked home-made cookies can bring back childhood memories for some people

- Hearing a song they used to hear at some emotional time can often take people back to a time or place, along with wonderful feelings and memories for many people

- Sights and sounds and smells of holidays often bring back delightful feelings

And a few unpleasant anchors:

- The bored and empty feeling that sends you rushing to the kitchen for comfort food

- The stress of not having enough time or feeling overworked makes you reach for food to deal with the stress upsets that cause you to reach for comfort food

- Certain songs like "Amazing Grace" that are often played at funerals can bring back feelings of sadness

Since we know that anchors are being created all the time, we can create our own anchors to create good feelings that empower us. The only reason you eat when you are not hungry is because of the feeling you get from it. Now you are going to create an anchor that you can use to feel even better than food and it has no calories.

An anchor can involve any of your five senses. You can use any combination of your senses to make the anchor more powerful. One of my favorite anchors for feeling good instead of eating, is a deep breath.

Right now, think of a time when you felt very happy. It could be any time that was recent or sometime in the past. As you think about this time, actually take yourself back to the time and place. See the people and the surroundings. Notice the sights, sounds, smells and anything that helps bring back the feeling. Now, make the feeling stronger and more intense. Close your eyes if necessary.

As you feel the feeling as strong as you can, take a nice deep breath and create the image of the perfect you, looking exactly as you want to be. As you exhale, feel a wonderful feeling of peace and calmness. Then say out loud, "Awesome" (or any other key word or phrase that you like).

Now, think of another time when you felt really happy. Repeat the process of making the feeling intense. Bring back the image of you and anchor it to a deep breath. Say out loud, "Awesome". Now, repeat this process at least one more time. The more you anchor it, the stronger it will become.

Now that you have a strong anchor, you are ready to use it. Imagine that you see one of the foods that you would normally eat too much of. Notice how you have a desire for this food. Now, take a nice deep breath and bring back those wonderful feelings with that image of the perfect you. As you exhale, feel a wonderful feeling of peace and calmness. Then say out loud, "Awesome". Notice how your desire for that food just seems to disappear.

Keys to powerful anchoring:

1. Anchor a very intense state such as a strongly felt experience.
2. Pick an experience that is unique, not mixed with other feelings.
3. Use unique anchors so the state is not mixed with a common action (like clasping your hands together).
4. Timing is important. Create the anchors just before the peak feeling and release it as the peak declines.
5. Reinforce the anchor. Every time you connect another experience to an anchor it becomes stronger.

*Every time you use your anchor or even your key word, it becomes stronger.

The Swish Pattern

When you create associations with food, there is often a trigger that stimulates the desire. For some people it may be a time or place. One woman I worked with had a desire for donuts every time she drove by a certain donut shop. Another person said that she would snack every afternoon when she went to the break room at work. After a few repetitions of association, it becomes like Ivan Pavlov and his dogs. He would ring a bell when he gave them food. After doing this several times, all he had to do was ring the bell and they would salivate.

One mental tool for making a behavioral change more automatic and consistent is the swish pattern. With the swish pattern, you identify the old behavior you want to change and the trigger that drives this behavior. Then you identify the new behavior you want to install. You mentally see the trigger and swish the old pattern with the new one.

The process is basically like this:

1. Identify the old behavior and the trigger that stimulates it.
2. Create a new feeling or behavior that you want to have.
3. Associate that with the trigger and have it replace the old mental picture.

Let's walk through the steps for the swish pattern:

First, identify the new behavior you want to have or the new feeling you want. Create an intense, fully disassociated internal representation of the new behavior that is desired. Being disassociated means you are watching yourself as though you are another person. Imagine yourself as the person you intend to be. See yourself as already being trim and healthy. Imagine how great it feels to be in control and no longer have food control you. Imagine the pleasure you would feel from the new behavior. Then take that picture and shrink it down to a little square in the bottom of your mind's eye. I like to imagine it like a computer screen when you have an icon at the bottom of the screen. When you click on the icon, it explodes and takes over the screen.

Make a big, bright picture of the old behavior. Be fully associated with the mental picture and feeling of the behavior to be changed, including the pain you feel from the behavior. Being associated means to experience the behavior and see it through your own eyes. Make this a moving picture that starts just before the trigger that creates your old behavior.

Notice exactly what the trigger is and when it appears in your movie. For the person who ate donuts, she imagined driving down the street where the donut store was located. The trigger was when the store came into view. For the person that snacked on her work break, it was necessary to identify what told her it was time to go on break. She said she went on break at 3:00pm every day. I asked how she knew it was 3:00. Was it a clock, a word from a coworker or some other signal? She said it was her digital desk clock as it turned to 3:00.

Once you have identified the trigger and the new behavior or feeling, simply swish the two pictures in your mind so that the old behavior automatically triggers the new behavior. The swish itself is done as follows:

Make a small, dark picture of the new behavior in the lower right-hand corner of the first picture, like a computer icon. Then run a movie that takes you to the time or place that you eat. When you see the trigger, have the new picture explode through the old behavior. In less than one second, simultaneously and enthusiastically, say the word "swish" or "yes" (or any work that creates excitement for you) and have the small picture explode in size and brightness until it bursts through the big picture just like clicking an icon on your computer. Pause to experience the new state fully.

Open your eyes or think of a blue sky with puffy white clouds to break the state and free your mind. This will allow you to go back and repeat the experience again rather than making it seems like one long experience.

Close your eyes and repeat the same steps again, at least five to ten times. Speed and repetition are keys to the success of the swish pattern.

If the old behavior pattern appears again, repeat the steps with ten to twenty repetitions. If you have done this correctly, the next time you see your trigger it will automatically bring up your new image with feelings.

Compulsion Blowout

This is a wonderful process developed by Richard Bundler, one of the creators of NLP. It takes only a few minutes to do and will have lasting effects.

Identify the compulsion you want to change – What is a food you absolutely have trouble staying away from?

Next, identify a food that you enjoy, but do not have a compulsion to eat.

Close your eyes and see, hear and feel the first food that you are addicted to. Experience this food to the fullest. Notice how you see the food. Notice how big the picture is. Is it close or far away? How bright is it? Is it in color or black and white? Is it moving? Notice how you experience it. What self talk is going through your mind? Are you saying things like, "I've got to have this food"? What feelings do you notice in your body? Where are they located? What is the intensity?

Now, open your eyes and let your body relax. Imagine a blue sky with puffy white clouds.

Close your eyes again and think about the second food. This is the food you enjoy without a compulsion to eat it. Notice how you see the food. Notice how big the picture is. Is it close or far away? How bright is it? Is it in color or black and white? Is it moving? Notice how you experience it. What self-talk is going through your mind? What feelings do you notice in your body? Where are they located? What is the intensity?

Now write down what you experienced for the first food and then the second. What was different between the two? Was there a difference in size, color, vividness, motion, feelings, self-talk, or anything else? Notice all the differences between the two experiences. Now, write down all of the differences you noticed.

Pick one difference that you noticed between the two and exaggerate it in the compulsive food. For example, if you noticed that the first food was bigger than the second, bring back the experience of the first food and keep making it bigger and bigger and bigger and notice your reaction to making it bigger. Notice how the experience changes.

If the self-talk was different, go back to the self-talk and make it more expressive. You might even make it sound more excited when you say, "I've got to have it!"

Perhaps the feeling was different. If the first food gave you a warm tingling feeling in your stomach, make it warmer and make the tingling feeling excite your stomach.

Repeat this with every difference that you found and notice how the experience changes for you. Notice which one of these differences is the strongest. This is the one that is the driving force of your compulsion.

Now, take the strong, driving force and blow it out. If the driving force was the size and brightness, make it bigger and brighter and bigger and brighter until it is blown out of proportion. Make it just overwhelming. Now think about how you feel about that food. If you still have some feelings of compulsion, repeat the blowout several times.

Then take the next one and do the same thing. If it is the voice, make it louder and more intense. Keep doing it until it is just shouting at you. Test it to see how you feel. Repeat this until the feeling has changed.

For a wrap-up of Chapter 5 go to http://www.emotionaldiet.com/review.html.

Chapter Six

Power Affirmations

"Whatever the mind of man can conceive and believe, it can achieve"
-Napoleon Hill

Affirmations have been a part of change for a long time, with mixed results. Some people will tell you their life changed with affirmations, while others will recite their affirmations until they are exhausted and nothing happens. So, what is the difference? In some cases, it is the way people write and think about their affirmations. More often it is the way most people recite their affirmations.

Let's try an exercise right now to point out what I mean. Sit in a quiet, relaxed state and say in a quiet voice, "I feel terrific". How does that feel? If you are like most people, you didn't feel very much. When I have people do this in seminars, only a few people will say that they actually feel a change. Most people will say they don't feel any different after saying that affirmation.

Now, let's try something different. Stand up in a confident stance with good posture. Make a powerful movement with your arms as you say the affirmation again. You might even want to shake your fist. Say the affirmation at the same time with emotion and feeling. Really say it as though you mean it – almost like you are shouting it out. Do this all together - scream, "I feel terrific!", as you shake your fist in the air.

Did you notice the difference? If you really did say it with feeling, while making a powerful gesture, you felt a surge of electricity going through your body. Your body is made up of energy – electricity to be exact. When you have a thought, like picking something up, your mind sends four volts of electricity through your muscles to your hand and creates the movement. When you make a quick, powerful movement, it creates a surge of energy through your body. When you add the feeling to the affirmation, along with the movement, it connects to your nervous system. This gives your affirmations incredible power.

> ## Energy + Motion = E-Motion

Power Affirmations are based on the following principles:
- Your present behavior is a direct result of your thoughts and feelings
- If you change how you feel, your behavior changes
- Power Affirmations change your feelings through your nervous system

To obtain maximum results from doing affirmations, there are certain guidelines that you should follow. Here are some suggestions to help you fire up your affirmations:

State Your Affirmation in Present Tense
Affirmations are more effective when they are stated in the present tense. For example; "I now have total control over the way I eat." Avoid affirming something in the future tense, such as, "I am going to have control over the way I eat", or the results will always be waiting to happen. I suggest creating affirmations that are directed at behavior, rather than outcome. Your subconscious may not believe you are already at your ideal weight, but it will believe you have the behavior of eating healthy food and exercising.

Be Positive
Create affirmations in the most positive terms that you can; avoid negative statements. Affirm what you do want, rather than what you do not want. For example; "I don't want to eat ice cream." This is a negative statement. A better affirmation would be, "I am now enjoying feeling good about my life without ice cream." The statement is as powerful as it is positive and it reinforces your desired goal.

Make them Short & Specific
Short affirmations are easy to say, and have a far greater impact on the subconscious mind, than those that are long and wordy. Keep them specific and to the point to add power and clarity. Your mind likes simple, direct concepts.

Repetition

Perhaps the single, greatest key to success with affirmations is repetition. That is what really imprints the affirmations into your subconscious mind. It is not the number of days you repeat the affirmations as much as the number of repetitions. Repeating a power affirmation ten times in one day will have almost the same effects as saying it once every day for ten days.

Emotion

Get involved, be passionate and use your emotions. Think carefully about the meaning of the words as you repeat them, rather than saying them passively. Energy + Motion = E-Motion

Belief

You don't necessarily have to believe your affirmations, initially. In fact, power affirmations are one of the fastest ways to change your limiting beliefs. They should be things that you know are possible. If you are 250 pounds and you say, "I am now 150 pounds", your subconscious mind may not buy it. Focus on your behavior with phrases like, "I love eating healthy foods in smaller amounts" or "I am now enjoying my trim, healthy body". Be sure to include affirmations that make you feel good now such as, "I am awesome" or "I feel powerful".

Make Them Your Own

Your affirmations must feel right for you. The more specific they are for your life and situation, the deeper the impression they make on your mind and the sooner you will experience positive results.

Energy + Motion = E-Motion
Affirmations by themselves have limited effect on change. To create change quickly, you need emotion. The easiest way to do this is to add motion to your affirmations with quick movements and strong feelings.

Write some of your affirmations to help you create the changes you want to create. One suggestion to make them personal and present is to start many of them with the words "I" or "I am now _____".

Example: "I now enjoy eating fresh fruits and vegetables".
             "I am now enjoying daily exercise".
             "I am now in total control of food and what I eat".
             "I am awesome! I am powerful! I am strong!"

_____

_____

_____

_____

_____

_____

_____

_____

_____

Start every morning with your power affirmations. The best time is right after your visualization exercise with your Blueprint For Success. It only takes a minute to create amazing changes in your beliefs and behavior.

As I mentioned before, the key to success with affirmations is the emotional feelings that you add to them. You can also have great success by sitting in a relaxed state and really creating the feeling of having already achieved the result you want. You will see an example of this in a later chapter on self hypnosis.

Affirmation Prayer

Prayer can give you the power to connect with a power that is greater than yourself. If you believe in a higher power, whatever you believe that power to be, allow that power to help guide you.

There are two types of prayers that are used to ask for what you want. One is to beg for what you don't have. That rarely works because you are acknowledging that you don't have what you want, reinforcing the thought that something is missing. The other way is to thank God (or the universe or whoever you pray to) in the present tense for something that seems to be in the future. For example: "Thank you God for my perfect health".

Say your affirmation prayer with a feeling of gratitude and state your desire as though you already have it. Feel those feelings of gratitude, joy and love of the higher power as you say it and feel what it will feel like to have what you desire. The power of your affirmation prayer is in the emotion. Repeat your affirmation prayer several times throughout the day, especially when you have a negative thought.

Here is an example of an affirmation prayer:

Thank you God for this trim and healthy body.
Thank you God for the joy of this day.
Thank you God for releasing me from the past and guiding me to my desires.
I love you God and I love myself.

Quiet Affirmations

Using quiet affirmations is a bit like affirmation prayer in the fact that you don't have to make a quick physical movement to be effective for you. What you do have to do is create the feelings that make the real emotional connection. Affirmations without feelings are just words. When you add the feelings to the affirmations, magic can happen.

Find a nice quiet place to sit and relax. Think about what you are grateful for. Create a positive feeling before you begin. You don't want to try to force the affirmations. You want to connect with the feeling and meaning of the words.

No matter how you choose to use your affirmations, the keys are repetition and emotion. Say your affirmations every day, even several times per day. Make this part of your daily routine and you will be amazed at the way your life begins to change.

For a wrap-up of Chapter 6 go to http://www.emotionaldiet.com/review.html.

Chapter Seven

Emotional Freedom Techniques

Any emotion, if it is sincere, is involuntary.
~Mark Twain

We have said, many times, that we are not driven by logic, we are driven by emotion. What if there was a way to release that emotional need?

Think how great it would be to instantly let go of stress, worry, emotional pain and the desire to eat when you are not hungry. Now there is a way to do just that. I am about to introduce you to what I believe it the most powerful way there is to be free of those emotional needs that drive you to eat.

This wonderfully effective and easy to use process is called Emotional Freedom Techniques or simply EFT. EFT is part of a growing field of health processes that target the body's energy system.

Everything in your body is made of energy. Eastern medicine has based much of its healing practice on the body's energy and the mind-body connection. Western medicine is just now starting to embrace the practices of eastern medicine and some American doctors have proclaimed energy healing as the next frontier in medicine.

Many therapists are now using energy therapy with very impressive results. It has become my favorite because it is so fast and effective in most cases. I have not experienced any adverse side effects in the hundreds of clients who have used this technique. One of the best features is that it is easy for anyone to learn and use. The more you use it, the more effective it can be. Experienced therapists who are able to uncover emotional issues can have fantastic results. More and more therapists are using energy therapy to compliment traditional therapy.

EFT uses some of the energy meridians that are used in acupuncture. In some ways, you could think of this as emotional acupuncture. Instead of using needles, you tap lightly on the energy meridians with your fingertips as you focus on the emotional issue that you want to resolve. So, what does that have to do with eating? As we've said before, we are not driven by logic, we are driven by emotions.

When I work with people for weight loss, I always ask them when they tend to overeat. I usually hear things like, "When I'm frustrated", "When I'm angry", "When I'm lonely", "When I'm bored", and the list goes on and on. These are all emotions. This tool will help you release those emotional drivers and take control of your life.

This book will give you the basics of using EFT for weight related issues. The EFT Process was developed by Gary Craig. He developed and refined the process based on Dr. Roger Callahan's process called Thought Field Therapy (TFT) which is also based on using the body's energy meridians. I have had the pleasure of attending Gary Craig's training classes and the results are truly impressive. He is a wonderful humanitarian who is truly focused on helping people. Many other experts have contributed to the further development of using EFT for almost any issue with an emotional component.

The science behind EFT is easy to understand. Your body has energy pathways called meridians that control the bioelectromagnetic energy flow. When you have an emotional disturbance, it can cause a disruption in the energy flow. One good example of this is stress. When you feel stressed, your body will tense up, sometimes creating muscle pain, headaches and other physical symptoms. Acupuncture has been shown to relieve many of these physical symptoms by restoring the energy flow. This is done by inserting tiny needles at the appropriate energy meridians. Acupuncture should only be performed by qualified practitioners with proper training.

EFT uses some of the same energy meridians to address emotional needs. When you feel a strong feeling, particularly a negative one, it causes a disruption in the energy flow. Instead of inserting tiny needles, you simply tap on the energy meridians with two fingers while focusing on the feeling.

When I work with individuals for weight issues, I find that the key to lasting success is to identify the emotional need they are trying to fulfill with food. Sometimes the feeling is easy to identify. For example, if they are bored, I just ask them what causes them to feel bored. If they say their job, their life or something about their life, it really means that something they desire is missing from their life. The next step is to identify what is missing and then find out why they are not doing something to fill that need. In the end, we identify the fear or other feeling that is holding them back and release that emotion. It is really amazing to see the changes that can occur in a person in such a short time when your remove the blocks that are holding them back.

In many ways, this is the same type of process that a therapist uses to identify an emotional issue that someone might be dealing with. I'm not suggesting that you need a therapist to deal with your eating, unless you have a serious eating disorder. It is my belief that just about everyone has some memories or feelings that keep them from having the most fulfilling life possible. When you eat to satisfy some hidden (or obvious) emotional need, you are missing some of the happiness you deserve and using food to try to make you happy. This technique will help you create happiness and a trim, healthy body.

One of the first questions I will ask a client with weight issues is, "Was there a time when you didn't have any weight issues?" Think back to your own life now and ask yourself that question. If the person says "Yes", I ask them if there was a time when they gained weight very quickly. If I get another "Yes", chances are that an emotional event happened at that time and is still affecting them.

Often people think that because an event happened long ago, it no longer affects them. To the subconscious mind, a memory is like a current event. The easiest way to identify this is to think of an emotional event from the past. If you remember it and still feel some of the same feelings, it is still affecting you.

I worked with one young woman I'll call Mary (not her real name), who was twenty-two years old at the time, and was about one hundred pounds overweight. I asked her if there had been a time when she gained weight suddenly and she said it started in high school at the age of seventeen. I asked her to just allow her mind to take her back to that time and to tell me what was going on in her life.

Mary said her parents were going through a really messy divorce. She described it as "the worst time of her life". When I asked her how it felt to think about it now, she still had many painful memories. These included feelings of hurt, betrayal, shame, guilt and loss. We tapped for each of these feelings and released all of the painful feelings from those memories. This doesn't change your memories, only the feelings attached to the memories.

I met with Mary one more time to work on these issues and her need for food disappeared. In addition to that, she started exercising and taking better care of herself because she felt good about herself and her life.

Sometimes the event that caused this feeling may not be apparent. If that is the case, just tap for the feeling you have and raise your awareness of that feeling. Allow your mind to just wander back to an earlier time when you may have felt that feeling. It may not come to you right away. It may even come to you when you are relaxed and thinking about something else.

Many people will remember a time when they were a child and dismiss that as not affecting them because they were so young. It is important to understand that the feelings attached to that event were those of a child who may not have been capable of logically internalizing those feelings. That means you are still dealing with the memory, using the feelings of a child. If you remember any memory and still feel some emotion about the event, it is still affecting you. Just close your eyes and allow yourself to relive the event as though you were a child again. When you feel the feelings getting stronger, measure the intensity and tap for the feelings until they lose the intensity. Then continue reliving the event until you release all of the emotion.

Some people may recall a feeling without an individual event. If you grew up feeling deprived or unloved and now use food to compensate, focus on the feelings as though you were back at that time. Then forgive anyone involved, including you, for holding on to these feelings.

Using EFT is actually very easy. A novice without any training can usually have success about 50% of the time. As you use it more, you will probably find your success rate going up every time. Experienced EFT practitioners often have a success rate of 90% or more.

You start by identifying the feeling you are experiencing. If you have a desire to eat when you are not hungry, notice exactly what you desire. Chances are, it is not fruits and vegetables. Then rate your feelings or anxiety on a scale of 0 (no anxiety) to 10 (uncontrollable urges and feelings).

Begin the EFT process by performing the set-up. You do this by tapping on the bottom edge of your hand between the fingers and wrist. This is called the karate chop point. As you tap with the first two fingers of your other hand, use the set-up phrase which has an affirmation, saying that having this desire does not make you a bad person. An example would be, "Even though I have this desire to eat this candy bar, I deeply and completely accept myself". Repeat this phrase three times while continuing to tap on the karate chop point.

Then tap 7 to 10 times on the remaining points with a shortened reminder phrase that keeps you focused on the feeling. An example would be, "This desire for this candy bar".

The remaining points are:
- **Top of the head** - right in the center
- **Eyebrow point** - where your eye brow meets the bridge of your nose
- **Side of the eye** - just outside of the eye socket
- **Under the eye** - at the top of the cheek bone
- **Under the nose** - between the nose and upper lip
- **Chin point** - between the lower lip and the chin
- **Collar bone** - right below your neck on either side
- **Side point** - about four inches under your arm pit

Repeat this sequence until the desire is either gone or at a manageable state. Then, focus on the real feeling that is causing this desire to eat. For example, you may feel bored, angry, frustrated, depressed or any number of feelings. You may even feel a combination of several feelings. If you feel more than one, address them one at a time starting with the one you feel the strongest. Then address each of the others in the order that they feel the strongest. This may seem like it will take a long time, but it really only takes a few minutes. Isn't it worth a few minutes of time for a lifetime of freedom? You know it is.

The key to being successful is to find the underlying cause of the feeling. This should be as specific as possible. For example, if you said you were feeling hurt you might say, "Even though I'm feeling hurt, I deeply and completely accept myself". This would address the emotion, however, you can increase your success by being more specific and identifying the cause of this hurt. You might say, "Even though I feel hurt because of the remark that Kim made about me, I deeply and completely accept myself". Notice that, in this case, you are focused on the feeling and not the person. You can't do anything about how someone else behaves, but you can do something about your own feelings. In a sense, you are taking ownership of your feelings instead of letting someone else push your buttons.

Many people find tremendous power by adding an additional part to the phrase, stating that they choose to feel differently. This was popularized by Dr. Pat Carrington. An example of this might be, "Even though I feel hurt because of the remark that Kim made about me, I deeply and completely accept myself and I now choose to let go of any remaining hurt". Another example might be, "I now choose to forgive Kim for this remark and move on".

Now that you have a basic idea of how EFT works, you can get started using it. The following pages have pictures and examples of the tapping points followed by some of the more common themes that show up with weight issues. Some of these are limiting beliefs that you can collapse with EFT as well.

Another important thing to do is be proactive. I start every day with a sequence of EFT for having an excellent day. During the day, I tap for being trim and healthy. I finish every night with a round of EFT for having a happy life. You will see examples of this on the following pages. For more information on EFT and its many applications, explore the section on EFT at http://www.emotionaldiet.com. To watch a video demonstration of EFT, go to http://www.emotionaldiet.com/review.html.

If you look at different EFT practitioners, you will probably find some slight variations. Gary Craig has even varied his process from what he used in his early training. Some of these may even vary depending on what issue you are working on.

One variation I use with weight and eating issues is in the set up phrase. Part of the phrase I use is, "I deeply and completely love and accept myself". The variation here is adding the word "love". Most people with eating issues have not really learned to love themselves. I have even had some people say they feel uncomfortable saying that part of the phrase. If you notice that feeling, ask yourself where that feeling came from. Go back to your list of things you like about yourself and read it every day. Find things to appreciate about yourself and others and you will find more joy in your life and less pain.

. *The basics of using EFT*

Focus on the feeling or emotion. Be as specific as possible.

Rate your anxiety or emotion. Decide how much it effects you on a scale of 0-10 (where 0 = no distress and 10 = highest level of feeling) when you think about it right now. How anxious are you? How uncomfortable do you feel?

Perform the Set-Up:
The Set-Up: While tapping on the Karate Chop Point, name the issue you have chosen to work on, followed by an affirmation about yourself.

Say it aloud with feeling.

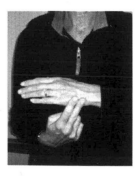

For example, let's say you have a craving for chocolate. You rate your desire at an 8 on a scale of 0 to 10.

Your setup:

"Even though I have this strong craving for chocolate, I deeply and completely love and accept myself."

While you are tapping on this Karate Chop Point, say your affirmation out loud 3 times. After you have completed this step, choose an easy, short reminder phrase to focus on the problem you want to work on, such as *"this anxiety desire for chocolate."*

TAP the energy meridian points as shown below. Start on the top of your head and work your way down. As you tap on each point in sequence, state your Reminder Phrase, such as *"this desire for chocolate."*

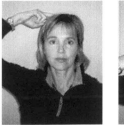

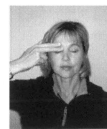

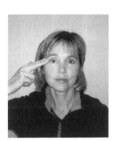

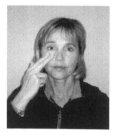

| Top of Head | Inside Eyebrow | Outside Eye | Under Eye |

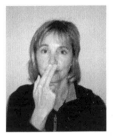

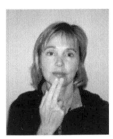

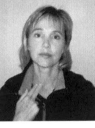

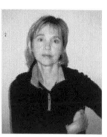

| Above Upper Lip | Chin | Collarbone | Side – 4" down |

Take a slow, deep breath and hold it for a second. Release it slowly through your mouth, allowing your anxiety to release with the breath.

Rate your anxiety or stress again.
Now think about the same problem again, and rate how you feel about it now on the 0 -10 point scale (10 means you really feel strong emotion, while 0 means it doesn't bother you at all).

Perform the Set-Up again.
Sometimes the stress or emotional feeling will be released with one round. Other times you may find that it is reduced but still there. If there is still some anxiety associated with the issue, repeat the same steps again. For example, suppose you rated your anxiety about your chocolate craving as a 7 on the 0-10 point scale, and after the first round of EFT, your craving dropped to a 4. You can continue tapping until you feel no anxiety or craving at all or the craving stays at a 1 or 2.

Revise your set-up statement to show that you have reduced some of the anxiety, but there is still more to work on.

An example of your modified set-up statement might be:

"Even though I still have some remaining cravings for chocolate, I deeply and completely love and accept myself."

TAP the stress-relief points again.
Go back and tap on all of the points while using a revised reminder phrase such as *"remaining cravings"* or *"remaining anxiety."*

Here is the basic process I like to follow using EFT for eating:

1. **Tap for the cravings or desire**

2. **Tap for the current emotional feelings driving the desire to eat**

3. **Tap for additional emotional feelings that appear**

4. **Use EFT to create positive feelings**

Let's take a look at how we might use each of those.

Tap away the cravings. Let's try this right now. If you have an unhealthy food handy that you often eat to excess, go grab it right now. I know what you are thinking – how silly is this to tempt myself with the very type of food I want to give up? Just stay with me and I think you will love the result. If you don't have any tempting food handy, just think of an unhealthy food that you often crave and allow yourself to create a desire for it right now.

Now that you have that food in front of you or in your mind, think how good it would taste to take a big bite of it right now. Really let your desire climb as high as you can. Smell the aroma and just think how much you would enjoy the guilty pleasure of that food right now.

On a scale of 1 to 10, how would you rate your desire at this moment? If it is only about 3 or 4 and you can't get it any higher, it is probably because you have been working on changing your behavior and you have lost some of your desire for this type of food. If this is something for which you still have a strong desire, it is probably because you have a strong emotional connection to it. You have either turned to it as a source of comfort or you have associated immense pleasure to it. Whatever your number is, see if you can make it as desirable as possible for this exercise.

Now we are going to perform the set-up. Use whatever food you have chosen in place of the example we use here. As you tap on the karate chop point with the first two fingers, say your set-up phrase out loud with feeling and emotion. To release the emotion associated with your eating or your feelings, it is very important to first get connected to that emotion. Let's say that you have a strong desire for cookies right now. Maybe you would rate your desire at 8 on a scale of 0 to 10. You would begin tapping the karate chop point while saying, *"Even though I have this desire for this cookie, I deeply and completely love and accept myself"*.

Be sure to say it like you really mean it. It helps the process if you say it strong enough to connect to that emotion. Repeat the set-up phrase two more times while tapping on the karate chop point.

Now tap on each of the other points about 7 to 10 times while repeating a short reminder phrase that keeps you focused on that feeling. Start on the top of the head and work your way down. The order is not really important, but most people find it easier to remember by going from top to bottom. In this case your reminder phrase might be, *"This desire for cookies"*. Repeat the phrase with every tapping point.

At the end, take a nice deep breath and slowly exhale through your mouth. Notice how relaxed you feel. Rate yourself on a scale of 0 to 10 and see where you are now. You will probably notice that your desire has decreased considerably. Let's say that you went down to 3.

Repeat the same process with a modified set-up. Now you would say something like, *"Even though I still have some remaining desire for this cookie, I deeply and completely love and accept myself"*. You are acknowledging that there is still some desire and also that the desire has decreased. Tap on the other points with a new reminder phrase such as, *"This remaining desire"*. Be sure to focus on that desire and notice how it has declined. At the end, take a nice deep breath and exhale slowly through your mouth. Rate yourself on a scale of 0 to 10 and see where you are now.

If you are at a 0, you can just walk away from that cookie with no problem. If you are at 1 or 2 (or higher), keep tapping until the desire is gone or you are at a low enough number that you don't need this cookie.

If you find that the tapping hasn't changed your feelings (this is rare), it is probably due to one of two things – either you didn't use enough emotion in the set-up to connect to the feeling or you are dehydrated. This process is based on the energy system in your body and water is the best conductor of electricity in your body..

Address the current emotional drivers for eating. We said that much of our eating is emotionally driven. Let's say that you are near a deadline at work and you are feeling some stress. The more you focus on the deadline, the more it bothers you. You want to do something to feel better and your first thought is food. It's not because you are hungry, it is because you want to relieve that feeling of stress. Basically, food becomes a distracter to take your mind off the issue that is causing the stress.

The problem is that after you eat the food, the problem that caused the stress still exists. Now you are mad at yourself for eating, so you have compounded the problem. EFT to the rescue!

First, tap for the desire to eat like we just talked about. After you have reduced your craving down to a 0 or the point where you don't need it, focus on the real cause of your stress. We said you are feeling the stress because of a deadline for work. Now you can tap for that feeling. Be as specific as possible. Instead of saying *"Even though I feel this stress"*, use a set-up phrase like *"Even though I feel stressed because I'm not ready for this deadline..."* Then you might follow it up with something else specific like, *"Even though I'm afraid of slowing down the project, if I don't make this deadline...".*

103

You'll notice that we used the word "afraid" in this set-up. Stress is really a code word for fear. When you say you are stressed, it is because you are afraid of something that may happen in the future. The more you focus on the fear of that event, the higher your stress level goes. Be as clear as you can on the real feeling that is showing up. Often, you will experience more than one emotion. If that happens, tap for the strongest one first and then tap for any remaining emotions.

It is important to follow up on your driving emotions for two reasons. First, the emotion is usually what is really behind your desire to eat. If you don't deal with the emotions, you are fixing the problem without addressing the cause. Secondly, the stress you are feeling causes your body to produce a chemical called cortisol which causes your body to store more fat.

Higher and more prolonged levels of cortisol in the bloodstream (like those associated with chronic stress) have been shown to have negative effects, such as:

- Increased abdominal fat, which is associated with a greater amount of health problems than fat deposited in other areas of the body

- Suppressed thyroid function, which can cause weight gain

- Imbalances in blood sugar

- Loss of bone density

- Loss of muscle tissue

- Higher blood pressure

- Lowered immunity and inflammation

- Impaired physical performance

For some people, the emotional desire is tied to their past experiences. I mentioned before that we usually associate cake to celebrations. When you connect the good feelings of a celebration to the cake, eating the cake brings back those good feelings. For those types of associations, using EFT one or two times will generally be enough to eliminate that association and you can look at the cake for what it really is – flour, sugar and other ingredients that you wouldn't care to eat alone.

Sometimes the association goes much deeper. For many years I had an uncontrollable urge to eat ice cream every night. No matter how full I was, I would still eat the ice cream, often having second helpings. It was not a habit, it was an obsession. Even when I was uncomfortable, I couldn't stop. I would just keep eating until I felt so bad that my stomach hurt.

Through hypnosis, (and the help of a fellow hypnotist) I was able to trace the source back to my childhood. My mother loved to have her ice cream every night, and I would always eat it with her. When she died, this became my physical connection to her, and that is when I developed the urge to eat ice cream every night. It was not the ice cream I desired. It was the feeling that I had associated to ice cream because of my memories of my mother.

I often ask people when they feel the urge to overeat. They usually say things like, "When I'm lonely, when I'm angry, when I'm depressed, when I'm bored" and countless other similar situations. Of course, these are all emotions that are driving this desire. Often these emotions have ties to past experiences that they are not even aware are still bothering them. There is an old expression, "Time heals all wounds". It may seem that way, but what usually happens, is that we just suppress these unresolved issues and we aren't even aware that they are still affecting us. If you can think of an event in the past and still feel emotions, it is still affecting you.

When you tap for the feelings that are driving you to eat, tune into those feelings and let them guide you back to earlier times when you felt those same feelings. Often the memory of an event from long ago will pop into your head. If it does, think back to that event and notice what feelings you are experiencing. Observe how high those feelings are and tap for them until they are down to zero or at least manageable. If you don't notice any memories showing up, that is fine. They may show up later or the next time you feel this emotion.

Look For and Address the Following Emotional Themes

Deprivation: *"Even though I feel deeply deprived...and I'm insatiable..."*

Abandonment: *"Even though I feel hurt about being abandoned..."*

Loss: *"Even though I feel indescribable losses inside..."*

Loneliness/ Emptiness: *"Even though I feel completely empty inside..."*

Anxiety: *"Even though I can't stop feeling anxious/ can't control my anxiety..."*

Guilt: *"Even though I suffer from too much guilt..."*

Fear: *"Even though I'm profoundly afraid..."*

Anger: *"Even though I can't stop feeling angry..."*

This list was created by Dr. Carol Look, who is an expert in using EFT for addictions. You can find her overeating protocol on Gary Craig's web site at http://www.emofree.com/addictions/compulsiveovereating.htm.

When I work with someone, I often have them tap for each of these themes, even if they say the feelings are not an issue.

For example, I worked with one woman for weight issues and I had her go through each of the emotions and just feel the feeling as if they were really strong right now. When we got to loss, she said that we could skip that one because there was nothing missing from her life and she had everything she could ask for.

I asked her to just focus on what it would feel if she had a loss and we started tapping. Suddenly she just stopped and a feeling of panic came to her face. I asked her what just popped into her mind and she told me about how her adult child had disappeared a few years before and was missing for several weeks.

She said that she thought she had left it in the past, but now that feeling was still strong. We tapped for the feeling and then I had her remember all of the events associated with the disappearance. We tapped for each one until there were no more feelings of loss. She felt a great feeling of relief. When I saw her a month later, she had lost 20 pounds and no longer had the emotional desire to eat.

Creating Emotional Freedom

The key to real success is going beyond tapping for cravings and finding the emotions and feelings that are really behind your emotional eating. Until you find and address these feelings, you are simply putting on a band-aid. You are addressing the immediate need but you are not really getting to the cause.

The following pages have some common feelings that many people experience. Go through each one as many times as you feel necessary to become free of emotional eating. Each one is a different issue that many people attach to eating.

You will go through three variations of the set-up phrase followed by one round of tapping on the negative feeling and a second round of positive feelings. Change the words, if necessary to make them work for you. Remember to take a deep breath at the end of the second round. As you go through these feelings, notice any other feelings that you experience. When you feel them, tap for all aspects of those feelings and any memories that surround them.

Release from Past Failures

Set-Up: Say Each Line While Tapping on Karate Chop Point

Even though I've never been able to lose weight in the past, I deeply and completely accept myself

Even though I feel like I've failed in the past, I deeply and completely accept myself

Even though I've felt disappointed in the past, I deeply and completely accept myself and I acknowledge my effort for trying

Round #1: Negative Reminder Phrases

Top of Head *I've never been able to lose weight*

Eyebrow *I feel like I've failed*

Side of Eye *I can't stick to a diet*

Under Eye *I've never made it long term*

Under Nose *I feel so disappointed*

Chin *Others can lose weight but I can't*

Collar Bone *No one else has ever failed*

Under Arm *There must be something wrong with me*

Round #2: Positive Phrases

Top of Head *There is nothing wrong with me*

Eyebrow *I was just doing it wrong*

Side of Eye *I had the wrong approach*

Under Eye *I don't need to diet*

Under Nose *I am a success*

Chin *I learn from the past*

Collar Bone *I am always growing*

Under Arm *I am amazing*

I Don't Believe I Can Change

Set-Up: Say Each Line While Tapping on Karate Chop Point

Even though I don't believe I can change, I deeply and completely accept myself

Even though I feel like I'm stuck in a rut, I deeply and completely accept myself

Even though I'm afraid I'll always be the same, I deeply and completely accept myself and I now allow myself to become the person I want to be

Round #1: Negative Reminder Phrases

Top of Head   *I've never been able to change*

Eyebrow   *I feel like I'm stuck*

Side of Eye   *I'll never be any different*

Under Eye   *I'll always be this way*

Under Nose   *No one has ever changed*

Chin   *It's just too hard for me to change*

Collar Bone   *I can't see myself differently*

Under Arm   *This is all I'll ever be*

Round #2: Positive Phrases

Top of Head   *Everybody changes*

Eyebrow   *I have changed lots of things in my life*

Side of Eye   *I've just been afraid it would be too hard*

Under Eye   *Maybe it's harder to stay the same*

Under Nose   *Maybe I need to change*

Chin   *I think I'm ready to change*

Collar Bone   *I welcome change*

Under Arm   *I love the new me*

I'll Always Be Heavy

Set-Up: Say Each Line While Tapping on Karate Chop Point

Even though I believe I'll always be heavy, I deeply and completely accept myself

Even though I feel like I was meant to be heavy, I deeply and completely accept myself

Even though It seems like it's just my nature to be heavy, I deeply and completely accept myself and I accept my body

Round #1: Negative Reminder Phrases

Top of Head	*I'll always be heavy*
Eyebrow	*I could never be thin*
Side of Eye	*Other people can be thin but not me*
Under Eye	*I guess I'm not like other people*
Under Nose	*I have no choice - I was born with big genes*
Chin	*My heavy genes make me eat, even if I don't want to*
Collar Bone	*Someone else got my skinny genes*
Under Arm	*I guess I'll have to be heavy whether I want to or not*

Round #2: Positive Phrases

Top of Head	*Maybe there is nothing wrong with my genes*
Eyebrow	*Maybe I've just used that as an excuse*
Side of Eye	*Maybe I do have a choice*
Under Eye	*I can choose to eat less*
Under Nose	*I can choose to exercise more*
Chin	*I can choose to be trim and healthy*
Collar Bone	*I love being trim and healthy*
Under Arm	*I love my new skinny genes*

I Don't Deserve to be Thin

Set-Up: Say Each Line While Tapping on Karate Chop Point

Even though I believe I don't deserve to be thin, I deeply and completely accept myself

Even though I feel like I'm not worthy of reaching my goal, I deeply and completely accept myself

Even though I feel I don't deserve to be trim and healthy because I somehow feel I haven't earned it, I deeply and completely accept myself

Round #1: Negative Reminder Phrases

Top of Head *I don't deserve to be thin*

Eyebrow *I'm not good enough to be thin*

Side of Eye *Other people deserve it more than me*

Under Eye *I'm just not worth that much*

Under Nose *I'm not important enough to be thin*

Chin *I haven't earned the right to be thin*

Collar Bone *Thin people are better than me*

Under Arm *I don't deserve to be like them*

Round #2: Positive Phrases

Top of Head *I am a special person*

Eyebrow *There is no one like me in the world*

Side of Eye *I deserve to be happy*

Under Eye *I deserve to be healthy*

Under Nose *I deserve to be trim*

Chin *I love myself*

Collar Bone *I am totally unique and special*

Under Arm *I deserve to be trim and healthy*

I'm Afraid to Let Go of This Problem

Set-Up: Say Each Line While Tapping on Karate Chop Point

Even though I'm afraid to let go of this problem (use your problem if you can), I deeply and completely accept myself

Even though I feel like I need to keep this problem, I deeply and completely accept myself

Even though I've identified with this problem and I don't know what I'll do without it, I deeply and completely accept myself and all my problems

Round #1: Negative Reminder Phrases

Top of Head	*I'm afraid to let go of this problem*
Eyebrow	*This problem is a part of me*
Side of Eye	*I identify with this problem*
Under Eye	*I've never been able to let go of this problem*
Under Nose	*I'm afraid I'll feel all alone without this problem*
Chin	*I feel like I need this problem*
Collar Bone	*My life will be empty without this problem*
Under Arm	*I'm afraid to let this problem go right now*

Round #2: Positive Phrases

Top of Head	*I am tired of having this problem*
Eyebrow	*I don't need this problem anymore*
Side of Eye	*This problem has taken too much of my life*
Under Eye	*I'm ready to take back my life now*
Under Nose	*I can always find new problems if I need them*
Chin	*I'm ready to be free from this problem*
Collar Bone	*I don't want this problem in my life anymore*
Under Arm	*I now choose to let go of this problem*

I Obsess About Food

Set-Up: Say Each Line While Tapping on Karate Chop Point

Even though I'm obsessed with food, I deeply and completely accept myself

Even though I think about food all day long, I deeply and completely accept myself

Even though thinking about food makes me feel happy, I deeply and completely accept myself and I now choose to release this obsession

Round #1: Negative Reminder Phrases

Top of Head This obsession with food

Eyebrow I think about food all of the time

Side of Eye I can't stop thinking about food

Under Eye I never get a chance to think about anything else

Under Nose I feel like food is my life

Chin Maybe I don't have a life

Collar Bone I'm just too obsessed with food to have a real life

Under Arm Because I think about food all day long

Round #2: Positive Phrases

Top of Head Maybe I can have a life

Eyebrow Maybe I can have other things in my life

Side of Eye I have so many other things I want to think about

Under Eye I don't have time to think about food all day long

Under Nose I am ready to let go of this obsession

Chin It doesn't serve me anymore

Collar Bone I am free of this obsession

Under Arm I choose to be in control

I Feel Bad About Being Overweight

Set-Up: Say Each Line While Tapping on Karate Chop Point

Even though I'm ashamed of myself for being overweight, I deeply and completely accept myself

Even though I'm embarrassed about my body, I deeply and completely accept myself

Even though I feel like everyone looks at me because I'm fat, I deeply and completely accept myself and I accept my body right now

Round #1: Negative Reminder Phrases

Top of Head *I feel embarrassed about being overweight*

Eyebrow *I feel like everyone stares at me because I'm heavy*

Side of Eye *I feel like they judge me because I'm fat*

Under Eye *I can't hide my fat*

Under Nose *I'm embarrassed to be in this body*

Chin *I'm ashamed of what I've done to myself*

Collar Bone *I'm ashamed of what I've done to my body*

Under Arm *I feel so ashamed of myself for being overweight*

Round #2: Positive Phrases

Top of Head *I'm happy that I still have this body*

Eyebrow *I thank my body for taking care of me*

Side of Eye *I have so much to be thankful for*

Under Eye *I don't need to feel sorry for myself anymore*

Under Nose *I don't think people really care how I look*

Chin *They're more concerned about how they look*

Collar Bone *I feel good that I'm taking better care of my body*

Under Arm *I feel good about myself because I am a good person*

Using Food as a Substitute

Set-Up: Say Each Line While Tapping on Karate Chop Point

Even though I use food as entertainment to change the way I feel, I deeply and completely accept myself

Even though I use food to avoid thinking about my real feelings, I deeply and completely accept myself

Even though I use food to fill something that is missing in my life, I deeply and completely accept myself and I acknowledge my feelings

Round #1: Negative Reminder Phrases

Top of Head   *Using food to fill a void*

Eyebrow   *Turning to food for comfort*

Side of Eye   *Food has become my best friend*

Under Eye   *I need my good friend, food to take care of me*

Under Nose   *I don't want to face my real feelings*

Chin   *It's easier to just stuff myself with food*

Collar Bone   *I love food because it loves me back*

Under Arm   *I need that feeling that food gives me*

Round #2: Positive Phrases

Top of Head   *Maybe I don't need food to feel better*

Eyebrow   *I'm tired of using food to fix my problems*

Side of Eye   *Food does not fix anything, it makes it worse*

Under Eye   *I want to feel better without food*

Under Nose   *I do feel better now without food*

Chin   *I feel a wonderful sense of freedom*

Collar Bone   *I love feeling good without food*

Under Arm   *I love being trim and healthy*

115

I'm Afraid of What Will Happen If I Change

Set-Up: Say Each Line While Tapping on Karate Chop Point

Even though I'm afraid of what my life will be if I change, I deeply and completely accept myself

Even though I'm afraid some of my friends won't like me if I change, I deeply and completely accept myself

Even though my friends might resent my success if I change, I deeply and completely accept myself and I accept my fears

Round #1: Negative Reminder Phrases

Top of Head *I'm afraid to change*

Eyebrow *Maybe my friends won't like me if I change*

Side of Eye *They might think I'm different*

Under Eye *I might miss the "old me"*

Under Nose *People might expect too much of me*

Chin *They might treat me differently*

Collar Bone *I'm afraid to let go of the "old me"*

Under Arm *I'm afraid I won't be able to change*

Round #2: Positive Phrases

Top of Head *Everything changes*

Eyebrow *Changing my body does not change my mind*

Side of Eye *I will still be the same person*

Under Eye *I will be an even better friend*

Under Nose *I'm tired of living this way*

Chin *I'm ready to be the person I was meant to be*

Collar Bone *I am excited about changing*

Under Arm *I was born to be trim and healthy*

I'm Afraid I'll Still Be Unhappy

Set-Up: Say Each Line While Tapping on Karate Chop Point

Even though I'm afraid I'll still be unhappy if I lose weight, I deeply and completely accept myself

Even though I'm afraid of being disappointed if my life is still the same, I deeply and completely accept myself

Even if I never get over my weight problem, I deeply and completely accept myself and I now choose to be happy

Round #1: Negative Reminder Phrases

Top of Head *I'm afraid I'll still be unhappy*

Eyebrow *I'm afraid I still will not feel fulfilled*

Side of Eye *I might still feel the same*

Under Eye *I'm afraid I won't be happy if I lose weight*

Under Nose *I'm afraid of being disappointed*

Chin *What if this doesn't make me happy?*

Collar Bone *I might be changing for nothing*

Under Arm *This fear that I still won't be happy*

Round #2: Positive Phrases

Top of Head *I don't have to change to be happy*

Eyebrow *I can be happy right now*

Side of Eye *I can be happy at any weight*

Under Eye *I make my own happiness*

Under Nose *I choose to be happy now*

Chin *I choose to be happy later*

Collar Bone *I am grateful for everything in my life now*

Under Arm *I am amazing*

117

Fear of Being Deprived

Set-Up: Say Each Line While Tapping on Karate Chop Point

Even though I'm afraid I'll feel deprived, I deeply and completely accept myself

Even though I don't know what I'll do if I'm deprived, I deeply and completely accept myself

Even though I have this empty feeling inside, I deeply and completely love and accept myself and I know that I have plenty

Round #1: Negative Reminder Phrases

Top of Head *I have this craving because I feel deprived*

Eyebrow *My deprivation makes me crave food*

Side of Eye *I fill my deprivation with food*

Under Eye *I feel deprived and crave my favorite food*

Under Nose *I feel so deprived*

Chin *I'm afraid there won't be enough*

Collar Bone *There is never enough*

Under Arm *I'm afraid I'll miss something*

Round #2: Positive Phrases

Top of Head *There is always enough*

Eyebrow *I am enough*

Side of Eye *I feel good when I pass up food*

Under Eye *I no longer have a need to eat everything*

Under Nose *I love to leave some food on my plate*

Chin *I have all I need*

Collar Bone *I like the feeling of having less*

Under Arm *My body feels better with less*

Guilty About Wasting Food

Set-Up: Say Each Line While Tapping on Karate Chop Point

Even though I feel guilty about wasting food, I deeply and completely accept myself

Even though I need to eat food instead of throwing it away, I deeply and completely accept myself

Even though I've never been able to throw food away because wasting it is a sin, I deeply and completely accept myself

Round #1: Negative Reminder Phrases

Top of Head *I feel guilty about wasting food*

Eyebrow *It is wrong to waste food*

Side of Eye *I feel this need to eat food instead of throwing it away*

Under Eye *Food should not be wasted*

Under Nose *I can't throw it away*

Chin *I have to eat it instead*

Collar Bone *Even if I'm full, I have to eat it*

Under Arm *I feel guilty when I throw food away*

Round #2: Positive Phrases

Top of Head *There is no reason to feel guilty*

Eyebrow *Eating too much food is hard on my body*

Side of Eye *If I eat when I'm full, I'm still throwing it away*

Under Eye *I choose to throw away what I don't want*

Under Nose *Eating food I don't need is the real waste*

Chin *I choose to let go of this feeling of guilt*

Collar Bone *It no longer serves me to feel guilty about throwing away food*

Under Arm *I feel good about eating only what I need*

I Feel Ashamed

Set-Up: Say Each Line While Tapping on Karate Chop Point

Even though I feel ashamed because I can't stop overeating, I deeply and completely accept myself

Even though I feel like I've let myself down, I deeply and completely accept myself

Even though I'm ashamed because I'm not what I want to be, I deeply and completely accept myself and I acknowledge my effort for trying

Round #1: Negative Reminder Phrases

Top of Head   *I feel so ashamed of myself*

Eyebrow   *I feel so inadequate*

Side of Eye   *I feel ashamed of myself*

Under Eye   *I'm so disappointed in myself*

Under Nose   *I'm ashamed of so many things in my life*

Chin   *I'm ashamed of the way I've acted*

Collar Bone   *This feeling of shame*

Under Arm   *I'm so ashamed of the way I've acted*

Round #2: Positive Phrases

Top of Head   *There is nothing to be ashamed of*

Eyebrow   *I was just doing the best I could*

Side of Eye   *I know that I can do better now*

Under Eye   *I'm ready to release this shame*

Under Nose   *I am a worthwhile person*

Chin   *I feel good about myself*

Collar Bone   *I am proud of facing my issues*

Under Arm   *I deserve to feel good again*

I Eat When I Feel Lonely

Set-Up: Say Each Line While Tapping on Karate Chop Point

Even though I feel lonely inside, I deeply and completely accept myself

Even though I've used food to fill this feeling of loneliness, I deeply and completely accept myself

Even though I feel like food is my best friend when I'm lonely, I deeply and completely love and accept myself

Round #1: Negative Reminder Phrases

Top of Head   *I'm afraid I'll be lonely without my extra weight*

Eyebrow   *I feel like food is my best friend*

Side of Eye   *I'll be lost without my best friend*

Under Eye   *I feel like I am so alone*

Under Nose   *I feel lonely inside*

Chin   *I feel lonely and empty*

Collar Bone   *I'll be alone without food as my friend*

Under Arm   *I just feel so lonely inside*

Round #2: Positive Phrases

Top of Head   *Food is not my friend, it is only food*

Eyebrow   *Food is just nutrition for my body*

Side of Eye   *I choose to fill my life with what I need instead of food*

Under Eye   *I'm tired of using food to fill my loneliness*

Under Nose   *I am ready to let go of my feelings of loneliness*

Chin   *I choose to feel good about myself*

Collar Bone   *I choose to feel good about my life*

Under Arm   *I choose to take control of my life instead of food controlling me*

I Can't Imagine Myself at My Goal Weight

Set-Up: Say Each Line While Tapping on Karate Chop Point

Even though I can't imagine myself at my goal weight, I deeply and completely accept myself

Even though I feel like I'll never reach my goal, I deeply and completely accept myself

Even though it seems like I'm just dreaming, I deeply and completely accept myself and I realize that dreams can come true

Round #1: Negative Reminder Phrases

Top of Head   I can't imagine myself at my goal weight

Eyebrow   I feel like I'll never make it

Side of Eye   It's just not possible for me

Under Eye   I've never made it before

Under Nose   I probably can't make it now

Chin   Others can reach their goal weight but I can't

Collar Bone   No one else has ever failed

Under Arm   There must be something wrong with me

Round #2: Positive Phrases

Top of Head   There is nothing wrong with me

Eyebrow   I don't need to be at my goal weight to be happy

Side of Eye   I can reach my goal weight

Under Eye   I don't need to reach a certain weight to be successful

Under Nose   I am a success

Chin   I learn from the past

Collar Bone   I am always growing

Under Arm   I choose to be happy at any weight

I Hate My Body

Set-Up: Say Each Line While Tapping on Karate Chop Point

Even though I hate my body no matter what I weigh, I deeply and completely accept myself

Even though I feel the pressure to eat the right foods and have the perfect body, I deeply and completely accept myself

Even though I hate my body and I reject my body, I can now love myself and accept myself at any weight and any shape

Round #1: Negative Reminder Phrases

Top of Head *I hate my body*

Eyebrow *I hate the way my body looks*

Side of Eye *I don't like the way I feel in my body*

Under Eye *I wish I were different*

Under Nose *I wish I had a different body*

Chin *It isn't fair*

Collar Bone *Other people have better bodies*

Under Arm *I reject my body*

Round #2: Positive Phrases

Top of Head *There is nothing wrong with my body*

Eyebrow *I choose to accept my body*

Side of Eye *I love myself and I choose to love my body*

Under Eye *I want to take care of my body*

Under Nose *My body is mine and I now choose to take responsibility*

Chin *I can be happy with the body I have*

Collar Bone *I now let go of the need to be perfect*

Under Arm *I can be happy without being perfect*

I Feel Angry About the Trap I've Been In

Set-Up: Say Each Line While Tapping on Karate Chop Point

Even though I feel angry about the trap I've been in, I deeply and completely accept myself

Even though I feel angry because I haven't allowed myself to be the person I want to be, I deeply and completely accept myself

Even though I feel angry about how much of my life I've wasted obsessing about my weight, I deeply and completely accept myself and my life

Round #1: Negative Reminder Phrases

Top of Head *I feel angry about the trap I've been in*

Eyebrow *I feel sad about the time I've wasted*

Side of Eye *I've wasted so much of my life*

Under Eye *I still feel a little angry*

Under Nose *I feel so disappointed in myself*

Chin *I didn't deserve to feel this way*

Collar Bone *I wish I could have accepted myself*

Under Arm *I feel sad about the trap I've kept myself in*

Round #2: Positive Phrases

Top of Head *I now choose to let go of the past*

Eyebrow *I no longer live in the past*

Side of Eye *Every day is a new opportunity to be happy*

Under Eye *I now choose to be happy*

Under Nose *I accept my life and my body*

Chin *I learn from the past*

Collar Bone *I am always growing*

Under Arm *I am living an amazing life*

Now that you have a good idea of how to work on the core issues that are driving you to eat, it is time to use your own specific issues and feelings. In earlier chapters, you recorded those feelings that are affecting you. If you skipped these exercises, please go back and do them now. The key to finally creating freedom from food addictions is to address the core feelings and emotions that drive your behavior.

Now is your time to finally break free and take control of your feelings!

Breaking Bonds That Hold You Back

At the end of Chapter 1 you created your blueprint for success. Some people have a hard time really accepting their new behavior or beliefs. Go back and identify any of these and tap for any limits you feel.

Clearing Limiting Beliefs That Have Blocked Your Success

At the end of Chapter 2 you identified some limiting beliefs that have held you back. Go back to that list now and tap for each of those. It may be hard to measure your feelings on a scale to zero to ten, so be sure to create a lot of emotion when you say the set-up.

Addressing Old behaviors and Feelings

In Chapter 3 you identified Actions That Are Not You, Behaviors and Feelings, and Secondary Gain. Go back and tap for each of these that you identified.

Triggers and Feelings That Drive You to Eat

In Chapter 4 you identified your triggers and feelings that you experience when you overeat. You also used your eating record to identify triggers and emotional causes of overeating. Imagine yourself in each trigger situation and tap on everything you identified until you notice a shift in your feelings.

Using EFT for Reinforcement

It is important to use EFT for reinforcement even if you don't feel cravings at the time. If you wait until you are headed to the refrigerator because of a compulsive urge, you are halfway there and it is harder to get yourself to stop and tap. Be proactive and take control of your feelings before they get out of control.

Before eating a meal (and several times throughout the day)

Before you eat a meal or a snack, use the EFT procedure repeating the following phrase three times as you tap on the bottom of your hand.

"Even though I have made unhealthy choices in the past, I deeply and completely love and accept myself and I now choose to be trim and healthy".

Now tap on the remaining meridian points. As you tap, repeat the phrase *"Trim and Healthy"*

Close your eyes, take a deep breath, hold and exhale slowly through your mouth.

Following Self Hypnosis and Before Affirmations

After using your hypnosis or before saying your affirmations, use the same EFT procedure as before a meal repeating the previous phrase three times as you tap on the bottom of your hand.

For a wrap-up of Chapter 7 go to http://www.emotionaldiet.com/review.html.

Chapter Eight

Using Self Hypnosis

"We know what we are, but know not what we may be"
~ William Shakespeare ~

I have been using hypnosis to help people make changes for many years. The first hurdle is always explaining exactly what hypnosis is – and what it is not. First of all, hypnosis is not mind control. No one can make you do anything you don't want to do or anything that does not match your internal values. Some people have false beliefs about hypnosis because of television programs and comedy clubs that feature stage hypnotists.

People often ask me, "Are you going to make me bark like a dog or cluck like a chicken?" I explain to them that the people who do that in a comedy club volunteer to go up on the stage knowing that this is their chance to act silly and not be responsible for their actions. Most of these people will act the same way after a couple of drinks. This does not mean I'm against stage hypnosis shows. I have several friends who are stage hypnotists and they are also very good at helping people make serious changes in their lives.

One thing you should know is that all hypnosis is really self hypnosis. No one can hypnotize you against your will. The hypnotist is actually your guide to help you create changes at the subconscious level. Let me explain a little more about how the mind works.

Your conscious mind allows you to think about the present moment and make decisions based on facts and logical reasoning. It is often referred to as the critical factor. Young children don't develop this critical factor until the age of about six or seven. If you tell a five-year-old that the moon is made up of green cheese, she will probably believe you. An adult will know that is not true, and even if they didn't know, they would evaluate your statement and question it. The conscious mind also contains short term memory and willpower. People often feel like they have failed when they give into temptation because they don't have the willpower to resist. The truth is, willpower is not designed to

127

help you resist temptation. Willpower is like a shot of adrenaline that keeps you focused on something for a short time. It is not for long term changes.

Your habits, feelings and beliefs are what really drive your behavior. These are all stored in your subconscious mind. This is the vast sum of all of your life experiences. I have said before that we are not driven by logic, we are driven by emotion. Your emotions are all stored in the subconscious part of your mind with your feelings and beliefs. When you consciously try to change your eating habits with willpower, you may have short term success, but you still feel like it is such a struggle. Part of you wants to change, but part of you wants to keep eating the wrong foods. In the end, it is the subconscious part of your mind that usually wins. That's when you throw up your hands and say, "I guess I'll always be like this".

The key to making permanent change is to make changes at the subconscious level. That is the role of hypnosis. It allows you to create a very relaxed state in your conscious mind also gives you the ability to bypass the critical factor to get to the subconscious mind without evaluating the suggestions.

Another point that you should know, is that hypnosis is not sleep. It is actually the opposite of sleep. Hypnosis is a relaxed state of narrowed focus which allows you to block out other distractions.

You may be wondering if you can be hypnotized. The answer is yes, you probably can. In fact, hypnosis is a natural state that everyone goes into at some degree every day. Hypnosis occurs when you enter what is called the Alpha State of consciousness. This is between your normal waking state and when you sleep. You pass through the Alpha State twice each day when you go to sleep and when you wake up.

You probably also go into a light hypnotic trance state several times throughout the day. Have you ever caught yourself daydreaming or caught up in a really good movie or book? When you are in this state, you may not even notice what others are saying or what is going on around you. This is a light state of hypnosis.

Have you ever driven home or somewhere else and you were thinking about something so intently that you couldn't remember what you saw on the way? You were perfectly capable of driving and stopping when you needed to, but you were so focused on what you were thinking about that you blocked out other distractions. This was another example of hypnosis.

Some people feel uncomfortable with the word "hypnosis". It is also called other names like guided imagery or visualization. The key is to make it vivid and feel the outcome. Your subconscious mind cannot tell the difference between a real and vividly imagined event. All you are doing is reprogramming your subconscious mind to create the behavior you want.

There are many types of self hypnosis that you can use to make the same changes. Some are easier to use than others. This is my favorite type of self hypnosis because it is so easy and effective. All you have to do is relax and slowly read out loud. The more you use it, the more effective you become. One reason it is so effective is because you use the sound of your own voice. Another reason is because you are actively involved. The key is to really engage your imagination and not just read passively.

Self Hypnosis

Find a nice quite place where you can relax. Put yourself into a positive state by reading the list of things you like about yourself.
Think about the good things that happened to you during the day. Remember nice things you did for others and what others did for you.
Close your eyes for a moment and allow all tension to leave your body as you totally relax. Slowly open your eyes and begin reading the induction aloud in a slow, relaxed tone.
At the end of the induction, close your eyes and slowly count backward from ten to one, allowing your mind and body to relax more deeply with each number.
Slowly open your eyes, keeping that relaxed state, and begin reading aloud in a slow, relaxed tone. Close your eyes after each affirmation and allow yourself to imagine and feel the meaning until you are ready to go to the next one.

Induction

I now feel a quiet sense of peace and comfort, and I allow the sound of my own voice to soothe my mind and body, as I speak slowly and softly. I become more relaxed and peaceful with every word I say and every thought I feel. With each passing moment, I feel my body and mind becoming more at ease. My mind is becoming as quiet as a peaceful summer night's dream. As my mind becomes quiet and clear, I allow myself to relax more deeply as I read and speak. I imagine I am in a beautiful peaceful place, surrounded by trees on a quiet day. My mind is as clear and quiet as the clear blue sky. I am in a relaxing rocking chair, rocking back and forth, back and forth, back and forth. I look at a leaf on a tree, and it is caught by a gentle breeze, swaying back and forth, back and forth until it gently falls from the tree. I watch it slowly sway back and forth as it drifts down, down, down gently floating down. As I watch it drift down, my mind drifts peacefully down with it. Being in this place makes me feel so relaxed and so good about myself. I now close my eyes and count slowly from ten down to one, relaxing more with each number until I am totally relaxed.

Affirmations

I realize that I am constantly changing and growing.

I am becoming aware of the strength and abilities that I feel within me.

I have a feeling of confidence in my ability to become the person I have chosen to be.

I appreciate myself as I am and I do good and kind things for myself.

Whatever I say and whatever I do is said and done with complete confidence that I will be successful.

I am free from the past and today is a new opportunity to live as I choose to be.

I begin now to program my body and mind to become the trim, healthy person I desire.

My energy increases as I become leaner, and I feel stronger and more vital.

I feel stronger and more confident as I become leaner and healthier.

I am proud of myself and the way I look and feel.

I see myself walking proudly, confident in my leaner body, as I go about my day.

I feel good about myself and no longer need food to comfort me.

I am at peace and I feel a great love for myself.

Food can never take the place of the unconditional love and support that I give myself.

Food is fuel for my body. I no longer use food to entertain or reward myself.

I no longer eat when I am bored. I refuse to use food to compensate for anything that is missing in my life.

If I am unhappy about something in my life, I address the issue that is making me feel that way. I no longer use food to satisfy any other need or want.

I have a deep and sincere respect for myself and for my body.

I want to eat healthy foods in just the right amounts for good nutrition.

I look and feel so much better when I eat only healthy foods.

I feel a sense of self-love and self-respect when I choose to eat right.

I choose to control my life. I refuse to let food control me.

I eat only enough to feel satisfied. I feel proud when I leave extra food that I don't need.

I eat slowly and carefully, focusing on how good I look and feel and how good my life is.

I enjoy drinking clean, clear, refreshing water. Drinking water makes me feel refreshed and renewed.

Sugar and fatty foods have lost their appeal for me. I now have a love and desire for fruits, vegetables and lean healthy foods.

I imagine myself eating these healthy foods. As I eat, it tastes so fresh and good.

I enjoy the taste of healthy foods and I feel good as I eat them.

I enjoy exercising in a way that is just right for me.

I feel so good about myself when I exercise and take control of my life.

I can feel the change in my body and my mind with each passing day.

Each of these ideas is now making a deep and permanent impression on my subconscious mind, and each day of my daily life I become more and more aware of the powerful expression of these true concepts

And now, as I close my eyes, I allow these suggestions to grow and become a part of me, as I enjoy the wonderful feeling of being so alive.

Take as long as you feel you need, to really feel the suggestions and feel so good about yourself.

Use this self hypnosis or listen to the hypnosis session every day for at least 30 days and then once per week for reinforcement.

You can download a complete 20 minute hypnosis weight loss session at http://www.emotionaldiet.com/downloads.html.

For a wrap-up of Chapter 8 go to http://www.emotionaldiet.com/review.html.

Chapter Nine

Food Made Easy

"When you are through changing, you are through"
. ~Bruce Barton

What were we born to eat? Humans are very adaptable. We have learned how to change our environment, create amazing technology and create food that can stay on the shelf for years without spoiling. But is that the best for your body? What were you born to eat? Humans are omnivores (eating plants and meat). Most other meat eaters have pointed teeth for ripping flesh and a digestive system that can handle raw meat. Even domestic animals like dogs and cats will chase and eat mice and rabbits.

Think of the type of mammals that are the most like humans. There is one species that shares over ninety percent of our DNA makeup. Of course, that would be the ape family. Some scientific theories suggest that humans evolved from apes. So, what do apes eat? Actually, apes are also omnivores like humans, but they are primarily vegetarians. They have bodies very similar to humans but don't suffer from most human ailments like high blood pressure and cholesterol. You've probably been wondering why you never see apes in McDonalds!

I'm not saying that we all have to give up our favorite fillet on the grill. We have evolved and our tastes in food have changed. What I am suggesting is that we would be more healthy if our diets included more of what our bodies were meant to eat and less of the unnatural foods that have become such a big part of today's diet.

An easy way to do that is to think of the foods that we can digest without preparation. Basically, that would be fruits, vegetables, grains and some fish. For many of us, the idea of uncooked fish may not seem appealing. Actually, there is a name for this delicacy. It is called sushi.

Most people have gotten into the habit of cooking most of their vegetables. The truth is, some of these foods lose a lot of their vitamins when they are cooked or overcooked. There are some problems like indigestion, acid reflux and irritable bowel syndrome that may actually be reduced by eating more whole raw foods.

One of the main reasons some experts say we should be eating more raw food, is because it still contains "live" enzymes which seem to help the stomach with digestion. These are sometimes known as "cultured" foods. It appears that heating food above 118 degrees Fahrenheit (48 degrees Celsius) destroys these healthy little enzymes. This could damage the food enough that it loses some of its nutritional value. One good way to help your digestion is to end your meal with a salad instead of dessert. The raw vegetables in the salad will help your digestion.

If your diet has been mostly tacos and macaroni and cheese, your stomach may not quite be ready for a steady diet of raw vegetables. You may want to start with just a few raw veggies at first. You can also try cooking some of your vegetables by baking, simmering or steaming them to make them more digestible. The key is to strengthen your digestive system by eating more cultured foods. Another source of cultured food is yogurt. You may have noticed the words "live cultures" on the label. "Live cultures" are those friendly little enzymes that help your body.

One thing you should know is that some of the best veggies can give you gas problems, especially when you are not used to them. These include broccoli, cauliflower, cabbage, kale, collards and brussel sprouts. Your body will certainly let you know it. You may need a little time to adjust to diet changes.

Another reason for many people to eat raw vegetables is the taste. I've never been particularly fond of the taste of broccoli, spinach, cabbage and some other vegetables that are especially healthful. Most of these have wonderful health benefits and are important to have in your diet. Cooking seems to enhance the natural flavor and aroma. That is fine for the people that enjoy the taste.

If they are not at the top of your list for flavor, you can subdue the taste by eating them raw. By mixing them in a salad with dressing and your favorite condiments, you can still get the benefits of these nutritious nuggets. Of course, the dressing will add fat and calories to your diet, so go easy on the dressing. Even if you dip them in veggie dip or cheese, it is still much better than not eating them at all.

Fats – The Good, the Bad and the Ugly

For a long time, we were warned to eliminate fat from our diet. The fact is that we all need fats. Fats help your body absorb nutrients, maintaining cell structure and are actually an important part of a healthy diet. However, too much fat, or the wrong kind of fat, will contribute to weight gain, heart disease and certain types of cancer. Fats are not created equal. Some fats promote your health positively while some increase your risks of heart disease. The key is to replace bad fats with good fats in your diet.

Saturated Fats – The Bad

Saturated fats raise total blood cholesterol as well as LDL cholesterol (the bad cholesterol). Saturated fats are found primarily in animal products such as meat, dairy, eggs and seafood. Some plant foods such as coconut oil, palm oil and palm kernel oil can be high in saturated fats. These fats are usually solid at room temperature. Saturated fats will clog your arteries and raise your risk of heart disease. Avoid them as much as you possibly can.

Refined vegetable oils are also included in bad fats. These oils have been processed with high heat, which damages the oil and removes healthy nutrients.

Examples of Bad Fats - Saturated Fats

- Animal Fat(usually 4-legged)
- Bacon
- Butter
- Cream & cream cheese
- Fried chicken
- Ice cream
- Lard & cooking grease
- Palm & palm kernel oil

135

Trans Fats – The Ugly

Several years ago, scientists invented a way to alter or "hydrogenate" liquid vegetable oils for food production to provide longer shelf life. That seemed like a good thing at the time. This hydrogenation process creates trans-fatty acids which were added to many commercially packaged foods. They can also be found in many commercially fried foods such as french fries at some fast food chains and some other packaged foods such as microwave popcorn.

Basically, trans-fat is made when manufacturers add hydrogen molecules to vegetable oil, which is why the process is called hydrogenation. The more hydrogen that is injected, the more solid it will become at room temperature. For a long time it was thought that margarine was healthier than butter because it was made from vegetable oil. Actually, this now becomes a chemically altered food that is not designed for human or animal consumption.

Because trans-fats are an unnatural substance, our bodies don't know how to process them. They will build up and clog your arteries and cause premature aging. Trans-fat, like saturated fat and dietary cholesterol, raises the LDL (Lousy) cholesterol that increases your risk for heart disease.

The U.S. Food and Drug Administration's website states:

Consumers can know if a food contains trans fat by looking at the ingredient list on the food label. If the ingredient list includes the words "shortening," "partially hydrogenated vegetable oil" or "hydrogenated vegetable oil," the food contains trans fat. Because ingredients are listed in descending order of predominance, smaller amounts are present when the ingredient is close to the end of the list.

> *If you see the words "hydrogenated", "partially hydrogenated" or "shortening" in the ingredients, you shouldn't eat it.*

One thing to know is that when a label says ZERO TRANS FATS, you should still read the ingredients. If a product has less than ½ gram of trans fat per serving, the label can say zero trans fats. If the product is border-line, the manufacture can just make the serving size smaller until it has less than ½ gram per serving. **Always read the label**. For more on reading labels, visit the FDA web site at www.cfsan.fda.gov/label.html.

Examples of Ugly Fats - Trans Fats

- Hydrogenated/partially hydrogenated oils
- Margarine (stick)
- Nondairy creamers
- Shortening

This Nutrition Facts label shows 13 grams of fat, of which 5 grams are saturated fat. What are the other 8 grams? We see 2 grams of trans fat and no unsaturated fat. Unsaturated fat will not be on the label. Even though the unsaturated fats may be good for us, they are also higher in calories than carbohydrates and protein.

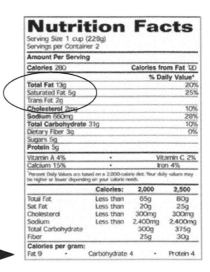

Unsaturated Fats – The Good

For a long time, we thought all fat was bad. Actually, there are good fats called unsaturated fats. These can actually help fight problems caused by the saturated fats. Unsaturated fats are found naturally in fish and plants that haven't been processed or damaged by high heat. These unsaturated fats come in two types – monounsaturated and polyunsaturated. The good news is that they both seem to be helpful in lowering cholesterol levels. Omega-3 fatty acids may actually help reverse clogged arteries.

Monounsaturated fats lower LDL cholesterol (the bad cholesterol) as well as total cholesterol and increase the HDL cholesterol (the good cholesterol). Foods such as nuts and plant oils like canola and olive oils are high in monounsaturated fats. It is important to realize that even with their health benefits; good fats are still higher in calories than protein and carbohydrates.

Examples of Monounsaturated Fat Foods

- Plant Oils (canola, olive, peanut, sesame)
- Olives
- Nuts – walnuts, almonds, peanuts, pistachios
- Peanut butter (non-hydrogenated)

Examples of Polyunsaturated Fat Foods

- Oil (corn, safflower, soybean, cottonseed)
- Salad dressing (regular & reduced-fat)
- Seeds (pumpkin, sunflower)

Omega-3 Fatty Acids

- Fatty cold-water fish such as salmon, cod, mackerel, tuna, herring
- Nuts & flaxseed

*Eating cold water fish like salmon once a week has been shown to lower heart disease by nearly 50%.

What Should I Eat?

For years we have had something called the Food Pyramid. At the bottom were the foods we should eat the most of, followed by the next kind of foods in smaller amounts as they went up the pyramid. One problem was that many foods were lumped together and it wasn't exactly accurate. The bottom line was that most people didn't follow it.

The FDA decided that it needed to be more clearly defined, so the food pyramid was redesigned into several pyramids. The result was that it became too complicated and again, most people didn't follow it.

What people need is something easy to use that makes sense. Here is the answer to that problem:

The Food Rectangle
(forget the pyramid)

Healthy Foods
Some Health Value
No Health Value
Unhealthy Foods

The Food Rectangle is based on an easy way to rate food. Basically, food comes in the following four categories:

Healthy Foods – The healthy food group contains only four types of foods in their natural state. Those foods are fruits, vegetables, whole grains and lean protein.

Some Health Value – These are primarily natural foods that are higher in natural fat or natural sugar. Examples of these are nuts, cheese, fruit juices and some dried fruits like raisins. The foods in this example contain important ingredients like protein, calcium and vitamins. They also tend to be higher in calories. The general rule here is: A little is good, a lot is not.

No Health Value – This is made up of foods that will not hurt you, but they don't help you either. If I could sum this category in one word, it would be "PROCESSED". It may have started as healthy food, but the good nutrition has been processed out of it. If the label says "Enriched", that just means that all of the vitamins and minerals were processed out and synthetic vitamins were added back in. This would be the same result as a small part of a vitamin pill.

> *In my opinion, this is the category that has created the overweight and obesity epidemic problem in America. Most highly processed foods have little natural value, are high on the glycemic index and raise your blood sugar quickly causing excess insulin release. These foods are not as filling and leave you hungry an hour later so you eat more. Examples of this would be most white bread, many cereals, instant potatoes, macaroni & cheese and almost any food that comes in a box.*

Unhealthy Foods – These are basically foods that have *no health value and are high in sugar, fat, sodium or chemicals*. If they have a combination of two or more of these ingredients, they are especially bad. Those are basically man-made foods that our bodies were not designed to handle. Common examples of this group are cookies, candy, soft drinks and most chips.

Rating Foods

Think about different foods as having a health value. Some foods have empty calories and no value at all. Some are actually unhealthy and harmful to your body. Some foods are very nutritious and healthy. And some foods have a limited amount of value.

Here is a scale to help us measure those categories:

0	2	4	6	8	10

Harmful   Empty Calories   Some Nutritional Value   Very Healthy

On a scale of zero through ten, list some of the foods that you feel would fall into each group. Some of these are probably foods that you have eaten in the past.

Very Healthy 7 - 10

1. _____
2. _____
3. _____
4. _____
5. _____

Some Nutritional Value 5 – 6

1. _____
2. _____
3. _____
4. _____
5. _____

Empty Calories (or very low value)   3 - 4

1. _____
2. _____
3. _____
4. _____
5. _____

Harmful   0 - 2

1. _____
2. _____
3. _____
4. _____
5. _____

You have probably already noticed that foods within a category are not all the same. For example, broccoli and potatoes are both vegetables in the healthy food group, but they are not equal in nutritional value. The broccoli has cancer fighting antioxidants while the potato has a lot of starch. Steak and sausage are both meats containing protein, but they are not the same nutritional value. What that means, is that we can put a food into a group quickly and easily, but we also need an easy way of comparing foods to each other.

Let's take another look at our rating scale.

0	2	4	6	8	10
Harmful	Empty Calories		Some Nutritional Value		Very Healthy

Think of a food that you believe would be at the top of the scale. Most people will say broccoli or blueberries because of the natural vitamins. Now think of a food that might be near the bottom. Many people will say cookies and chips because they both have a combination of fat and either sugar or salt.

The worst that I can remember someone saying was deep fat fried Twinkies. That really does sound bad. To begin with, Twinkies are not what I would call real food. They feel more like a real sponge than sponge cake, and that filling reminds me of something I would use to caulk my house. They have an incredibly long shelf life, which no natural food would have, so they are probably heavy in preservatives. When you deep fat fry them and they soak up trans fats, you have a recipe for clogged arteries and high blood pressure.

The way we use the ratings system is very easy. You start by putting the food in a category and then adjust it according to where you think it should be. For example, broccoli is at the top so we'll give it a ten. A banana does have some vitamins, although not as much so we'll give it an eight. Lean protein is in the healthy food group, but what if it isn't lean?

I saw an ad recently for hot dogs at 59 cents per pound. Just think - a whole pound of meat for only 59 cents! Let's look at what goes into hot dogs. Most hot dogs are made from leftover scraps of intestines and fat that would be discarded. By grinding them up and putting them into a long round shape with a skin on it, they not only avoid the expense of disposing of the scraps, they can make money from these waste products. They are incredibility high in fat and have cancer causing preservatives like sodium nitrite. It is not natural for any meat to last for three months.

Let's compare different types of meat, which is a good source of protein. Fish would probably be very high, especially if it has omega-3 fatty acids. We'll give salmon a ten. Turkey breast would be very good, so we'll give it a nine. Dark meat would be lower, maybe a seven or eight. Beef would probably be a little lower because red meat is higher in saturated fat. The more fat it has, the lower value we give it. If your hamburger is 93% lean, it would be higher than 84% lean, which would be higher than 70% lean. This does not have to be an exact science.

The more nutrients it has, the more you move it up the scale. The more fat, sugar, salt or preservatives it has, the more you move it down. It's that easy.

Now that you have an idea of how the Food Rectangle works, here is your goal for healthy eating:

> **- At least 50% of your food should come from the Healthy Food Group.**
>
> **- At least 80% of your food should have a rating of 5 or above**

It's that simple. When I introduced this at one of my seminars, a woman immediately spoke up and asked, "Does that mean I have to give up my meat and potatoes?" I said, "No, it means that you fill half of your plates with fruits and vegetables first and then put your meat and potatoes on the rest".

The typical meal usually looks something like this: a nice big steak, a mound of mashed potatoes and gravy and a token vegetable of three green beans. Plan your meals around the healthy foods. Make them your focus and make the rest extra. This doesn't mean that you can never eat cake again. Just get at least 50% from the healthy group and 80% with a rating of 5 or above.

I know that some experts will argue that everything should be healthy foods. Time for a reality check! When you feel deprived, you will crave foods you don't eat. If you just limit how much unhealthy food you eat, you can raise your quality of nutrition without feeling deprived. You may also find that as your tastes change, your desire for these unhealthy foods disappears.

The fact is many people find that most of their diet is closer to a 5 and below instead of a 5 and above. Let's take a look at America's favorite weekday lunch and see how it measures up. Can you guess what that meal might be? That's right! *A burger with fries and a soft drink*!

To measure this meal, we have to take each item separately. Let's start with the burger. Chances are you went to a fast food restaurant for this meal. Do you think they use the leanest hamburger? My guess is that they don't. This does have protein, but it also has more fat than we really want. It would fall into the Some Health Value group. Since it is higher in fat, we'll move it down toward the bottom of the group. Most people give it a rating of 5.

What did you top this burger with? If you got some veggies like lettuce, tomato and onions, that is a plus. Most people go with the basic pickle, ketchup and mustard. The pickle started as a vegetable, but it is now pickled in salt, so we would move it down to a 5. The ketchup started with tomatoes, but it is now full of sugar (processed). We could still give it a 4 or 5 because tomatoes retain lycopene, even when processed. Mustard has no food value and no calories.

We'll give it a 4 because it will not hurt you. Another favorite topping is cheese. Do you think that fast food restaurant uses real cheese or processed? My guess is processed. We'll give it a 4.

How about that bun? Do you think it is made with whole grain? No, because whole grain buns would cost more. That means it falls into the "No Food Value" group which is primarily processed food. It not only has the nutrients processed out, it will shoot up your blood sugar quicker than table sugar. We'll give it a 4.

Let's look at those fries. They started as a vegetable as well, although not a highly rated one. The problem is that they are fried in oil, some including trans fat, until all of the nutrition has been replaced with fat. Then they are topped with a lot of salt. Some restaurants will soak them in sugar to enhance the taste and help keep them firm when fried. So now we have something that has no food value that is loaded with sugar, salt and fat. How bad are they for you? Well, let me ask you this. Have you ever eaten fries in your car and accidentally dropped a couple of them under the seat? Six months later, while you are vacuuming the car you find them and you notice that they still look the same. They aren't rotten, they aren't moldy, and they haven't even fallen apart. In fact, they still look like they did the day you dropped them. Flies haven't bothered them, mice haven't eaten them, ants haven't eaten them, but this is what we eat. Obviously, these belong in the Unhealthy Food Group. We'll give them a 1.

What about that soft drink? To start with, we know it doesn't have any food value. If it has added sugar, it moves into the Unhealthy Food Group. OK, what about diet soft drinks? They don't have added sugar. If you have followed Aspartame (sold under the name of NutraSweet), you know that there are a lot of health concerns connected with it. I have talked to people who have noticed a big improvement in their health and concentration ability when they stopped drinking diet soft drinks. Even thought the FDA says it is safe, when something gets that much negative attention, I tend to stay away from it. I haven't heard as much negative feedback about sucralose (sold under the name of Splenda), so I tend to favor that. There are concerns about it as well, so I don't overdo it.

Any artificial sweetener will raise your desire for sweets.

One thing that you will find in that soft drink is carbonation. This will increase the acid level in your body and change your PH balance. Your body is like a swimming pool. You need to keep it balanced for good health. It would take 33 glasses of water to balance the effects of one glass of carbonated soda. The best we can give this soft drink is a 2.

Now, let's look back at our meal and see how close we came to our goal of 50% from the healthy food group and 80% with a rating of 5 and above. There was nothing from the healthy food group. We gave the hamburger patty a 5 along with the ketchup and pickle. Everything else was rated a 4 or less.

What You Ate Yesterday

Think back to everything you ate yesterday (or the past 24 hours). This should include all of your regular meals and any snacks you had. Even if it was just a handful of nuts or popcorn, write it down. List each food item separately.

Beside each food item, write down a point value for that food.

Food	**Value**

145

Now take a look at the values you have listed. How many were below 5? How many were above 5? How many were unhealthy (0 - 2)? How many were healthy (8 - 10)?

If you have way too many foods that are below 5, you really need to change what you are eating. Remember, it is not enough to be thinner. Your goal is to be trim and healthy. You can actually get to your ideal weight by eating junk food if you eat a small enough amount, but you wouldn't be healthy.

Moving Up the Food Chain

Many people have two main concerns about changing to a healthy diet:
1) They are afraid that it will be too drastic and they can't stick to it.
2) They are afraid that it will taste like cardboard and they will no longer enjoy eating.

This doesn't have to be a drastic change. Many people have started with whole milk, then switched to 2%, then 1% and finally ended up with non-fat milk. You don't have to go right from junk food to vegetarian. Your goal is to move up the scale to healthier foods. This is what I call "Moving up the food chain". If you are currently snacking on food with a rating of 4 and you switch to something rated at 6 you have made a healthy improvement.

Another reason is that you need to follow your desires until you create a stronger desire for healthy foods. It is as simple as this – when you want a cookie, there is no amount of celery that will satisfy that desire. What you need to do is identify the characteristics and find a healthier alternative that has those characteristics. Is the food hard or soft, hot or cold, sweet, sour or salty?

Let's say you have a desire for cookies. The characteristics are crunchy and sweet with a baked flavor. My favorite substitutes for cookies are the Quaker Oat Squares cereal or Honey Nut Shredded Wheat. They are made from whole grain, however they do have some added sugar and sodium. On a flavor scale, they are probably just a little below cookies.

On our eating scale, they are probably a 5 or 6 compared to cookies which would be a 1 or a 2. Remember, your tastes will change as you eat different foods and lose your desire for unhealthy food. I can't remember the last time I ate a cookie. I'm not saying I will never eat one again. What I am saying is that now when I think of a cookie, I imagine piles of sugar and lard that went into the cookie and I just don't have a desire for it. Just imagining the greasy, sugary texture in my mouth is a turn off for me.

Another common one is ice cream. It is cool, creamy and sweet. The most common reframe for ice cream is yogurt. The low-fat flavored yogurts are really delicious with only about 60 calories. They come in great flavors like apple pie, coconut crème and various fruits. I usually choose the brands that are flavored with Splenda (sucrose) because of all of the bad things I have read about NutraSweet (aspartame).

> ### *When you want a cookie, there is no amount of celery that will satisfy your desire!*

Of course, someone always asks me about chocolate. The truth is that there really is no substitute for chocolate. That doesn't mean you can't move up the food chain. Dark chocolate has been shown to be beneficial to your health. Another way to satisfy that chocolate urge is to have chocolate covered almonds, raisins, strawberries or other healthy food. Make your own chocolate dip. Remember to limit the amount you have because they still have calories.

You can use this process for any type of food that you eat. If you decide that yogurt will not satisfy your urge and you have to eat ice cream, you can still move up the food chain. First, have real ice cream that is made from natural ingredients like Breyer's. The fewer additives and chemicals you have, the better. Now, put half the amount of ice cream in your bowl that you would normally eat. Then top it off with fresh (or frozen) fruit like bananas, strawberries, blueberries, pineapple or whatever fruit you prefer. You might even throw on a few healthy nuts like almonds or walnuts. Remember, there are still calories, but this fruit sundae is much healthier than ice cream alone and it will satisfy that urge.

Some people are not sweet eaters but they do like salty snack foods like potato chips or cheese curls. Again, you can have the type of foods you enjoy and still move up the food chain. Start by looking at the ingredients on those chips you are eating. Avoid the ones that have a long list of ingredients, especially when you don't recognize them or can't pronounce them. Stick with the basics. When I buy chips, I look for ones that have only corn, vegetable oil and salt. Then I look for the brand with the lowest amount of salt and fat. Baked chips have less oil with fewer calories and fat. Then I get some of my favorite salsa. Most salsa is made from healthy ingredients like crushed tomatoes, peppers and primarily healthy foods. Again, look for the brand with low sodium.

Load up those chips with salsa and you will find you eat fewer chips and you can still satisfy that urge. Also remember that they still have calories. Eat them slowly and savor the flavor, knowing that you are making healthier choices.

One person I worked with had developed an addiction to smoothies. When I say addiction, remember that this is just something you do compulsively on a regular basis. You can become psychologically addicted to any type of food by creating associations. She knew the smoothies had about 350 calories, but she still had the urge to have one every day. We found a healthier alternative (and much less expensive) at the local grocery story. They had yogurt fruit smoothies that were only 70 calories and very delicious. I have to admit, I tried one myself and it was really good. She was able to satisfy that urge and still move up the food chain.

Be especially aware of canned food like chili, stew and other similar food items. Most of these are extremely high in sodium. Be sure to check the labels.

Make it a habit to try to move up the food chain at least one number with most of the foods you eat. When you are looking for healthier choices, start with the fewest and most natural ingredients you can find.

Reframing the Unhealthy Foods That You Eat to Excess

Write down 10 foods that you have a hard time passing up or that you eat too much. Identify the characteristics of the food, such as the texture, sweet or salty, soft or crunchy, etc. Then write down a healthy (or healthier) alternative food that is similar in characteristics.

Unhealthy Food   Healthy Alternative

1. _____   _____
2. _____   _____
3. _____   _____
4. _____   _____
5. _____   _____
6. _____   _____
7. _____   _____
8. _____   _____
9. _____   _____
10._____   _____

Every time you reach for some food, ask yourself this question:
"Is this going to help me or hurt me?"

"If man made it, don't eat it!"
- Jack LaLanne -

149

Daily Assignment

One of the most effective ways to guide you to change your eating habits is to keep a food diary. In Chapter 4, you have an emotional eating record. This will just record your feeling and not your food. If you want to, you can just include what kind of food you eat on that record. If you don't want to write everything down as you go, you can take a few minutes in the evening and write down what you ate. Be sure to write down a point value beside each item. Use one letter to identify the section of the food rectangle it is from. For example:

H = Healthy, S = Some Food Value, N = No Food Value and U = Unhealthy.

Your goal is to have at least 50% from the Healthy group (more is better) and at least 80% of your food should have a point value of 5 or above. If you have had an excess of unhealthy foods, take a minute and make those foods seem less attractive to you. Then make some healthy foods more attractive.

For a wrap-up of Chapter 9 go to http://www.emotionaldiet.com/review.html.

Chapter Ten

Your Healthy Body

The only difference between a rut and a grave is their dimensions.
~Ellen Glasgow

In America, one out of every two people dies of heart disease. Also, one out of every three dies of cancer. You might say that is because we are living longer, but heart disease and cancer are two of the more preventable diseases. So, what causes you to become ill? In a word, you can attribute most illness to one thing – the accumulation of toxins. Remember, there are more than just the physical toxins. Toxic emotions like fear, hate and stress can also weaken the body and immune system. We'll talk about those later.

When I work with smokers, I tell them that I really don't believe that smoking causes cancer. Actually, it probably does indirectly, but I don't believe it is the direct cause. Cancer is basically a disease of the immune system. We all have renegade cells called free radicals roaming around our bodies. When a healthy immune system detects these free radicals, it will destroy them before they can do any harm. When the immune system is weak, the free radicals gain strength, form tumors and spread through the body.

Cigarettes are very toxic. They release over four thousand chemicals including nicotine (very poisonous in concentrated form), DDT (used in rat poison) and formaldehyde (used in embalming). These are not a high enough level of poison to kill you right away, but the immune system of a smoker is constantly trying to recover from the constant stream of poison. That leaves the free radicals an opening to start taking control of your body. Smokers are not only more susceptible to cancer; they are more susceptible to almost every disease down to the common cold.

Eating toxic food will do the same thing. Foods laden with pesticides and chemicals put your body in a constant state of recovery and weaken your immune system. Your body is amazing in its ability to cope until you overdo it.

Many disorders including heart disease, diabetes, stroke and cancer have been found to be largely preventable. We are now realizing that even though the disease may come from the outside, as in a virus, the internal healing mechanism of the immune system is the most important healer.

The very best medicine is already in us. Our bodies are capable of natural good health if we just stop abusing them. We should also learn and apply methods to activate its ability to heal us. Research has shown that diet, exercise and stress management are powerful tools for maintaining health.

In the Western world we have a "quick-fix" mentality. A new diet craze shows up almost every day. Modern medicine is focused more on fixing diseases than preventing them. Self-care is one of the most important features of the Asian traditional systems of medicine. Most of these ancient philosophical and medical theories encourage the individual to take responsibility to maintain or enhance their health. By practicing some simple methods every day, you can boost your immune system and increase your energy and vitality.

Cells: The Basic Building Blocks of Life

Everything in your body is made up of one thing – cells. In fact, there are over 100 trillion cells in your body. Different parts of your body may react differently to the food you eat, but every part of your living body is made up of cells.

To be healthy, your cells need 3 things:
1. Oxygen - the source of life and energy in the body.
2. Necessary nutrients to stay healthy.
3. The ability to eliminate their own waste.

Now, imagine your body as one big cell. How would it feel if it was full of waste with no nutrition and very little oxygen? Your cells are calling out for help!

Oxygen – the Breath of Life

The most common killer of cells is lack of oxygen. Most people in the western world have become very shallow breathers. That means we use the top half of our lungs to bring in oxygen while the bottom half accumulates with unreleased excess carbon monoxide. This becomes a toxin in the body and inhibits good health.

Most people don't stop to consider the importance of proper breathing techniques. After all, we know how to breathe, don't we? It seems a little silly to put extra attention to something we do naturally. Notice your own breathing right now. Is each breath actually very shallow?

The lymph system is basically the sewage system of the body. There is not a built-in pump for the lymph. It is basically pumped through muscular movement. Deep breathing cleanses the lymph system and oxygenates the body. Dr. Jack Shield, who actually put microscopic cameras inside people's bodies, found that nothing stimulates the lymph system more than a deep diaphragm breath. It multiplies lymph flow ten to fifteen times more than normal.

When you change your volume and rate of breathing, some very dramatic physiological and even emotional changes can occur. According to recent studies, the lungs, diaphragm and thorax work together to form a pump for the lymph fluid, much like a heart pumps blood.

Hospital studies have shown the benefits of breathing exercises in the recovery of everything from surgery to the common cold. Patients who practice these forms of breathing daily will respond more quickly to treatment, no matter what type of treatment they are receiving. Individuals who are already healthy are able to reduce stress and retain good health when they practice deep breathing exercises daily.

I am a big fan of yoga for many reasons. It helps your body by strengthening the muscles, increasing flexibility, reducing stress with relaxation and teaching you controlled deep breathing. This is a modified form of yoga breathing.

153

Full Chest and Abdominal Breathing. This method is simply a controlled deepening of the breath. You inhale slowly for a count of four, then hold it for a count of four and exhale through your mouth for a count of six.

Start by taking a slow, deep, breath through the nose as you slowly count to four. When the diaphragm drops down, the abdomen is expanded allowing the air to rush into the vacuum created in the lungs. Then the chest cavity is expanded, allowing the lungs to fill completely.

Then hold it for a count of four as you constrict your abdomen. When you pull your abdomen in, you will feel the pressure in your lungs as it forces the oxygen into your cells, bloodstream and your brain. This can make you feel a bit light-headed and dizzy, so take it slow and easy at first and practice it sitting down. It is best to avoid doing this while driving or operating machinery.

Now exhale slowly through your mouth for a count of six or until all of the air is expelled from your lungs. When you do this, your next breath will fill your lungs with pure, rich oxygen.

To maintain good health, do 6 to 10 repetitions, 2 to 3 times per day. The most important time to do this is just before you go to bed. That is when your body recovers from physical and emotional demands. When you oxygenate your body before sleeping, you will eliminate toxins from your body which will allow it to recover faster. The deep breathing is also a great relaxation technique. Most people report more restful sleep right away.

The second best time to practice deep breathing is when you first get up in the morning. It will energize your body, revive your brain and increase your metabolism. Take a few minutes to relax and meditate when you first get up. Then take 10 deep power breaths.

Water – the River of Life

I remember watching an episode of the television program "Star Trek" in which an alien species used a weapon that basically removed all traces of water from the victim's body. All that remained was a small pile of minerals. There was nothing that resembled their former body. Sometimes science fiction will remind us of the science part that is based on reality.

Two thirds of your body is water. You have probably heard that before. The fluid that lives in your cells is made up of water. The blood that enriches your body is made up of water. Imagine what your dishes would be like if you never washed them. The food would get hard and crusty, start to build up and probably smell terrible. Your cells are the same way. Without water to flush away the waste, kidneys can't function, the immune system can't circulate and toxins will accumulate in your cells. The major cause of illness is a buildup of toxins in your system. The best way to flush toxins out of your cells is by drinking plenty of water. Doctors recommend that you drink more water when you are ill. In today's world of toxins in our food, drinks and air, we need to help our bodies all we can.

I grew up in farm country and I know that when there is a drought year, crops are stunted and weak. No matter how much fertilizer you put on the ground, without water, the fertilizer will never get to the roots and help the plants grow. Your body works much the same way. Water is the main transportation system for everything that circulates in your body. Without water, nutrients can't flow from your food to your muscles and brain.

One other way to eliminate toxins is through your pores. When you perspire, your body cools itself by releasing water through your skin. You can lose a quart of water through sweat if you exercise hard for an hour. If you are not hydrated, your body doesn't cool itself and you risk heat stroke or other heat related problems. Remember that everything we do depends on our cells functioning properly. If you want your cells to function at their peak (and who wants wimpy cells?) then you need to provide your body with enough water to do its job.

Right now you may be saying, "No problem, I drink lots of coffee and soft drinks". That is not the same as drinking plain water. In fact, drinks that contain caffeine can lead to dehydration. In one seminar, I mentioned the importance of plain water and one man told us about his teenage son who had been feeling constantly tired with very little energy. They suspected that he had mononucleosis and took him to their doctor for an examination. The doctor tested the young man and said he was suffering from chronic dehydration. "How can that be?" asked the puzzled teen, "I drink fifteen Mountain Dews every day!"

One of the most common causes of fatigue is dehydration. Your brain is about seventy-two percent water. If you have a three percent drop in the water level of your brain, it sends a signal to your body saying "I'm tired". If you try to fix the fatigue with coffee or cola, it's even worse. You burn up your remaining energy much faster and are left more dehydrated by the coffee, which is a diuretic. Often I hear someone say, "I don't know what is wrong with me today. I ate nutritious food and got plenty of sleep, but I'm so tired". When I hear this (or experience it myself) I always suggest a big glass of water. Within minutes, the fatigue is gone and energy is sky high again.

Sometimes people will mistake dehydration for hunger. They may feel like their blood sugar is low and have the urge to snack to raise their energy level. Drinking a glass of water before eating anything will often release that desire to eat and leave you feeling totally refreshed.

Another benefit of drinking water is that it speeds up your metabolism and burns more calories. This is especially true of cold water because your body burns energy to bring the temperature down.

Hot water is often referred to as "Chinese Penicillin" because of its healing ability. I like to alternate hot and cold water.

On the average, Americans drink more than 400 calories per day. Think about that. If you substituted water for those calories, you would drop nearly one pound every week without even giving up your favorite foods. That adds up to over forty pounds in one year! Recently I ran into someone who had been in one of my seminars for improving your mind power. I talk a lot about the importance of water and the effects dehydration has on the brain. This person had lost over twenty pounds and looked fantastic. She said that all she had done was switch from her usual drinks to water. That's all! No diets, no extra exercise, just lots of water.

* If you tend to drink a lot of sweetened drinks or fruit juices, you probably want to consider drinking less of that and more water.

How much is enough? One common formula is to divide your weight by two and drink that many ounces of water. If you weigh 120 pounds, that would be sixty ounces or just over seven eight-ounce glasses. To make it easier, I like to just suggest eight glasses of water every day. Another good source of water is to eat water-rich food such as fruits and vegetables. These "living waters" will enhance your skin as well as every part of your body.

Is all water the same? There are a lot of different opinions of water with studies and statistics to support them all. My feeling is, all water is good for you and some is better than others. Let's start with tap water. Tap water is perfectly safe in major cities of America and most major developed countries. Most of it has two chemicals that your body doesn't really need.

The first one is chlorine. Do you know what the main ingredient of bleach is? That's right, it is chlorine. It is also added to swimming pools to kill all of the extra bacteria from the bodies in the water. That is what creates the strong smell and makes your eyes burn. Chlorine is added to drinking water to kill bacteria because it has to travel through miles of underground pipes that are not exactly sterile. The amount of chlorine that is added to the water is perfectly safe for you to drink. All major cities constantly test their water to monitor the quality. It can affect the taste in some areas.

Another chemical that is often added to water is fluoride. This is supposed to reduce cavities in your teeth. Many scientists have questioned the value of fluoride in drinking water and the possible negative effects on your body. Again, both sides have studies and statistics to support their claims. Since I am not a scientist, here is my take on fluoride. It may help prevent cavities in enamel, but there is only one part of your body that contains enamel and that is your teeth. Most people gulp down their water without much of it really getting on their teeth. If you use toothpaste that contains fluoride, notice the warning label that is required to be on it. It will say something like, *"Warning - If you swallow more than used for brushing, call the Poison Control Center immediately"*. That doesn't exactly give me a warm and fuzzy feeling.

I'm not saying you shouldn't drink tap water. It is perfectly safe and your body is capable of filtering out these chemicals. At the same time, I can't see putting anything in my body that it doesn't need because it just creates more work to eliminate chemicals and toxins. My first choice is bottled water. Realize that just because it comes in a bottle doesn't mean it is any different than your tap. Some bottled water is right out of the tap and will say it is from a "municipal water source". Some bottles will say "filtered" which can mean a lot of different things. The best way to remove impurities is through reverse osmosis. It should say this right on the label.

One big reason to use bottled water is the taste. Some tap water will taste great while others will be pretty strong. Many opponents of bottled water do mention the environmental cost of plastic as well as the fact that tap water is free. That is a good point. Please be sure to recycle plastic bottles. I usually buy gallons of bottled water because it is much cheaper. I don't see any value in the more expensive types of water, but that is an individual choice.

Do not reuse small water bottles for more than one day. The bacteria will multiply on it, even though it is your bacteria. Most thin plastic used for bottled water is not meant to be washed. The soap and warm water can cause the plastic to break down. Use a heavy plastic or metal bottle for refilling.

Another good suggestion is to use a filter on your tap water at home. Even the inexpensive carbon filters will remove about ninety-seven percent of chlorine. If you prefer, you can get a pitcher with a filter that will do an excellent job and improve the taste of your water. A twist of lemon is also a great way to enhance the taste without calories.

Let me just say that there is nothing wrong with drinking tap water. It is much better than drinking other beverages and is certainly much better than being dehydrated. If you do drink tap water, take advantage of the added chemicals before you swallow. Swish it around in your mouth to get the fluoride on your teeth and let the chlorine reduce the bacteria in your mouth. Having healthy teeth and gums is important to good health, and the bacteria in your mouth can lead to bad breath.

Antioxidant Foods

We already know that some foods are healthier than others, but some are really health boosters for scavenging free radicals in your system. One way of measuring food value is called Oxygen Radical Absorbance Capacity, or ORAC. This measures the total antioxidant power of foods and is used regularly by the food and nutrition industries.

I've heard it said that we don't die, we just kill ourselves. Research suggests that eating plenty of high-ORAC foods may help slow the process of aging in both your body and brain. Foods that score high in ORAC antioxidant analysis may protect cells and their components from oxidative damage, according to ORAC studies at the USDA Agricultural Research Service's Human Nutrition Research Center on Aging at Tufts University in Boston.

According to research findings, High-ORAC foods can:

- Raise the antioxidant power of human blood 10 to 25 percent.

- Prevent some loss of long-term memory and learning ability.

- Maintain the ability of brain cells to respond to a chemical stimulus which normally decreases with age.

- Protect blood vessels and capillaries against oxygen damage

Top Antioxidant Foods (ORAC* units per 100 grams)

Fruits		Vegetables	
Prunes	5770	Kale	1770
Raisins	2830	Spinach	1260
Blueberries	2400	Brussels sprouts	980
Blackberries	2036	Alfalfa sprouts	930
Strawberries	1540	Broccoli florets	890
Raspberries	1220	Beets	840
Plums	949	Red bell peppers	710

159

Oranges	750	Onions	450
Red grapes	739	Corn	400
Cherries	670	Eggplant	390

Super Foods That Help Your Body

As we talked about earlier with the food rectangle, we want to get 50% of our food from the "Healthy" category. Not all foods are the same value in this category. Some foods have been identified at "Super Foods" that can boost your health and vitality. This term was first used in Dr. Steven Pratt's book, Super Foods Rx. Here are some of the top choices identified by Dr. Pratt and other leading researchers. Try to include some of these in your diet every day.

Beans - Before you start the jokes, realize that beans are a great combination of fiber and protein. This is the ideal protein source for vegans, and it helps you feel full longer and stabilize your blood sugar. Some great choices are Pinto, Navy, Lima, chickpeas.

Blueberries – Blueberries are at the top of the fruit sources. They taste great and they are very high in organic compounds called phytonutrients. Other good fruit sources are raspberries, strawberries, cherries and purple grapes.

Broccoli - Broccoli might be the best food you can eat. It is one of the best cancer fighters known. It's loaded with antioxidants and carotenoids to fight cancer, and the fiber can help with weight loss. You can get similar benefits from brussel sprouts, cabbage, kale, cauliflower, collards and mustard greens.

Fiber – Okay, this isn't really a specific food but rather a component of food. A diet high in fiber will help you maintain healthy cholesterol and blood sugar levels. Because fiber helps you feel full longer, it's a helps you curb your appetite. Whole grains, beans, fruit, and vegetables are all good sources. Fresh, frozen, or dried are the best. You can use canned fruits, but canned veggies tend to be higher in sodium.

Oatmeal - Steel cut oats are full of fiber and can lower your calorie needs for your next meal by 30%. They can also help lower cholesterol. Avoid the highly processed, high sugar oatmeal.

Omega 3-Rich Fish - Cold water fish like salmon is at the top of the list for protein. Omega-3 fatty acids can stabilize your blood sugar levels and help clear clogged arteries. Most cold water fish such as Alaskan halibut, sardines and trout are also high in Omega-3. Fish oil capsules are a great supplement.

Oranges - Fresh oranges contain pectin, which is a fiber that is found in citrus fruits. You can also find pectin grapefruit and tangerines. Fruit juice does not contain much fiber and does not provide this same benefit.

Pumpkin - This is actually squash, which is rich in carotenoids and fiber. Skip the pie crust and mix it with low fat cheese to makes a great low carb snack. Fresh steamed pumpkin is better than the canned pie filling. You might also try butternut squash.

Soy - Soy contains isoflavones, which can help prevent fat storage. Look for tofu, soy milk, or soy nuts -- not soy powder.

Spinach – Popeye was right. This is a high fiber super food that is also a natural source of iron. It is especially good for your eyes and can help prevent macular degeneration.

Tea - All teas are not created equal. The antioxidant power of black tea and green tea are far above herbal teas. Green tea also has a powerful antioxidant called ECGC. A Japanese study on green tea found that men who drank green tea regularly had lower cholesterol than those who didn't. Other studies have shown that ECGC can inhibit the growth of cancer cells. If you are not ready to give up your coffee, try mixing tea with your coffee in your drip coffee maker.

Tomatoes - Tomatoes are high in Vitamin C and help to naturally produce carnitine, an amino acid that helps you burn fat. They are also a great source of lycopene, especially when they are cooked.

Turkey - Turkey has 30% fewer calories and 50% less fat than beef. The white breast meat is best. You can get similar benefits from skinless chicken breast.

Walnuts - Walnuts are a great source of protein and Omega 3 fatty-acids. They are also low in carbs, but they do contain more calories. You can get similar benefits from almonds, pistachios, sesame seeds, peanuts, macadamia nuts, pecans, hazelnuts and cashews.

Tea - Try cutting back on your coffee and substitute a cup or two of tea. This drink has antioxidants and flavanoids, which can increase your metabolism. Either green or black teas are best. Herbal teas do not provide the same benefit.

Yogurt - Low-fat dairy has become the new "diet food", because it speeds up your fat burning metabolism and provides protein and calcium. Yogurt is especially good because it contains "live cultures", which are bacteria that help your intestines with digestion. My favorite desert is vanilla yogurt with fresh strawberries.

And Finally, the best Super food Yet ... Dark Chocolate – This could be the breakthrough everyone has been praying for. New research has shown that dark chocolate is loaded with antioxidants and can actually lower blood pressure. Before you run to the candy bar isle, realize that not all chocolate is the same. Look for chocolate with 60% or higher cocoa content; the darker, the better. In fact, the darker it is, the lower the fat and sugar content will be. Now that's our kind of health food!

The foods on list are from Dr. Pratt's book and other food experts. I have studied nutrition and physiology, but my real expertise is in human behavior. That is why I turn to experts in the health field for advice.

Anyone can search the internet and find information on any topic including health. I don't take anything I find as truth, just because it is on some web site. I usually look for two criteria when I research health information.

First, I look for someone who is actually in the medical field such as an MD or a registered dietitian. I mentioned MD here, but I have to clarify that being a doctor is not enough. To become a doctor requires very little in the way of nutritional study. Most doctors are trained to diagnose and fix problems instead of prevention. I look for doctors that are interested in preventing problems first.

The second thing I look for is being open to possibilities outside of the normal procedures. Many physicians limit their thinking to the standard procedures and refuse to accept anything outside of the narrow medical guidelines.

One of my favorites is Dr. Mehmet Oz, who is a regular guest on Oprah's television program. He does a great job of explaining medicine to mainstream people. He has often said that when something gets results, we should study it instead of judging it against the current accepted processes. Some of my other favorites are Dr. Michael Roizen, who created the Real Age program, and Dr. Andrew Weil, an American author and physician, best known for establishing and popularizing the field of integrative medicine.

What is the Glycemic Index?

I mentioned that the biggest problem in today's diet is the abundance of processed food. These are processed to the point that all of the natural nutrients are destroyed and usually replaced with high amounts of sodium and sugars. These simple sugars can cause a release in insulin which causes you to store fat around your middle.

Here is basically what happens in a simplified form. When you eat carbohydrates, your body breaks them down into glucose or blood sugar. This gives your body a steady supply of energy. Your cells have little receptors that monitor the amount of sugar in your bloodstream. If you have too much sugar in your blood, your blood will become thick and syrupy. To counteract this, your pancreas will release insulin to thin out your blood and allow it to flow better.

Overly processed food is in a simple unnatural form that causes wear and tear on the pancreas. Instead of being digested at a normal rate like complex sugars (also known as complex carbohydrates), simple sugars (which are processed carbohydrates such as white flour and processed natural sugars like corn syrup) immediately enter the bloodstream through the tiny capillaries in the intestinal walls without having to go through normal digestive channels. This causes an insulin rush, which is repeated every time you ingest simple sugars. This is what causes wear and tear on the pancreas, which was not designed to produce insulin at such enormous and rapid rates. The insulin is also responsible for causing your body to store fat around the middle, which is the most dangerous place to carry fat.

When you continue to eat too much simple-carbohydrate, highly-processed food, your pancreas gets overworked and the receptors become dulled. Then your body does not produce an adequate amount of insulin to thin your blood. The blood thickens and will not flow as well to the small capillaries in your eyes and extremities like your fingers and toes. The numbness in your fingers and blurred vision that occur are the first signs of type II diabetes.

It is important to know what types of foods break down quickly in the blood stream. One measurement of this is the glycemic index.

The glycemic index is a ranking of carbohydrates based on their immediate effect on blood glucose (blood sugar) levels. It compares the carbohydrates of different foods, gram for gram. Carbohydrates that break down quickly during digestion have the highest glycemic indexes. The blood glucose response to these foods is fast and high. Carbohydrates that break down slowly, releasing glucose gradually into the blood stream, have lower glycemic indexes.

Some advantages of eating a diet that is low on the Glycemic Index:
• Avoids a quick rise in blood sugar after eating
• Helps reduce body fat – especially around the middle
• Improves your body's sensitivity to insulin
• Helps control diabetes
• Helps you feel full longer
• Keeps your energy level up to stay physically active longer

Some simple ways to switch to a Low GI Diet:
• Eat more whole fruits and vegetables
• Eat cereals that contain oats, barley and bran
• Eat whole grain breads, pasta and cereals
• Reduce the amount of starchy foods like potatoes
• Eliminate processed foods
• Eat more salads with whole vegetables

To avoid blood sugar levels spikes, try eating five small meals per day and flavoring with high acidic vinegar and lemon which slows digestion. Another suggestion is to combine good fats and protein with your carbohydrates to slow absorption and avoid blood sugar spikes.

The following table will give you an example of the glycemic index of some common foods:

Under 55: Low   Between 55-70: Intermediate   Over 70: High

Glycemic Index Table

Beans		Breads	
baked	44	bagel, plain	72
black beans, boiled	30	baguette	95
butter, boiled	33	croissant	67
cannelloni beans	31	dark rye	76
garbanzo, boiled	34	hamburger bun	61
kidney, boiled	29	apple muffin	44
kidney, canned	52	cinnamon muffin	44
lentils, green, brown	30	blueberry muffin	59
lima, boiled	32	oat & raisin muffin	54
navy beans	38	pita	57
pinto, boiled	39	pizza, cheese	60
red lentils, boiled	27	pumpernickel	49
soy, boiled	16	sourdough	54
		rye	64
Cereals		white	70
All Bran	51	wheat	68
Bran Buds	45		
Bran Flakes	74	**Cereal Grains**	
Cheerios	74	barley	25
Corn Chex	83	basmati white rice	58
Cornflakes	83	bulgar	48
Cream of Wheat	66	couscous	65
Frosted Flakes	55	cornmeal	68
Grapenuts	67	millet	71
Life	66		
muesli, natural	54	**Crackers**	
Nutri-grain	66	graham	74

165

oatmeal	48	rice cakes	80
Puffed Wheat	67	rye	68
Raisin Bran	73	soda	72
Rice Chex	89	Wheat Thins	67
Shredded Wheat	67		
Special K	54	**Drinks**	
Total	76	apple juice	40
		colas	65

Fruit

		Gatorade	78
apple	38	grapefruit juice	48
apricots	57	orange juice	46
banana	56	pineapple juice	46
cantaloupe	65		
cherries	22	**Milk Products**	
dates	103	chocolate milk	35
grapefruit	25	custard	43
grapes	46	ice cream, van	60
kiwi	52	ice milk, van	50
mango	55	skim milk	32
orange	43	soy milk	31
papaya	58	tofu frozen dessert	115
peach	42	whole milk	30
pear	58	yogurt, fruit	36
pineapple	66	yogurt, plain	14
plums	39		
prunes	15	**Pasta**	
raisins	64	cheese tortellini	50
watermelon	72	fettuccini	32
		linguini	50

Root Crops

		macaroni	46
French fries / chips	75	spaghetti, 5 min boiled	33
pot, new, boiled	59	spaghetti, 15 min boiled	44
pot, red, baked	93	spaghetti, protein enrich	28
pot, sweet	52	vermicelli	35
pot, white, boiled	63		
pot, white, mash	70	**Snacks**	
yam	54	chocolate bar	49
		corn chips	72

166

Soups/Vegetables		croissant	67
beets, canned	64	doughnut	76
black bean soup	64	graham crackers	74
carrots, fresh, boil	49	jelly beans	80
corn, sweet	56	Life Savers	70
green pea, soup	66	oatmeal cookie	57
green pea, frozen	47	pizza, cheese & tom	60
lima beans, frozen	32	Pizza Hut, supreme	33
parsnips	97	popcorn, light micro	55
peas, fresh, boil	48	potato chips	56
split pea soup w/ham	66	pound cake	54
tomato soup	38	Power bars	58
		pretzels	83
Sugars		saltine crackers	74
fructose	22	shortbread cookies	64
honey	62	Snickers bar	41
maltose	105	strawberry jam	51
table sugar	64	vanilla wafers	77
		Wheat Thins	67

Perhaps the most in depth GI info available on the Internet at the moment is the Glycemic Index site (www.glycemicindex.com). Check out the database provided on this site to find GI values for all sorts of foods. The site has been put together by researchers at the University of Sydney.

Increase Your Brain Power

"Would you like to raise your IQ ten points by next week?" I teach a class at the local community college called "Double Your Mind Power" and I always start the first session with that question. Of course, everyone answers "yes". The truth is you actually can! The fastest and easiest way to improve your brainpower and help keep your mind sharp is to eat healthy. I spend the first class talking about nutrition and the effect it has on the human brain.

The brain is an organ, just like every other part of your body. When you eat a diet high in sugar, fat, chemicals and simple carbohydrates, your brain actually will not function as well. Once you give it proper nutrition, it will become more effective immediately.

The brain actually runs primarily on carbohydrates. When you go on a low-carb diet, you will find that you don't think as clearly and remember as well. Your thinking becomes a bit hazy and dulled. That is one reason I'm not fond of diets that eliminate most carbs.

On the other hand, eating simple sugars will cause a rise in insulin, which will then cause you to feel tired and listless and your brain will not operate at peak efficiency. There is probably no other organ in your body that will be affected by your diet as quickly or as much as your brain. Here are some ways that you can increase your brain power:

- Eat primarily fruits, vegetables and complex carbohydrates.
- Eat more beans and legumes.
- Eat nuts - walnuts and almonds are the best.
- Eat cold water fish which is high in omega-3 fats or take fish oil capsules.
- Cut out most animal fat. Eat lean meats and remove skin from poultry.
- Cut down on sodium and sugar.
- Eliminate trans fats.
- Eliminate most processed foods.

For more information on brain health, check out one of my favorite books on this topic called "Your Miracle Brain" by Jean Carper.

"The ability of a meal's composition to affect the production of brain chemicals distinguishes the brain from all other organs. The crucial compounds that regulate other organs are largely independent of whatever was in the last meal we ate - but not the brain."

- Richard Wurthman, research-psychiatrist, MIT -

For a wrap-up of Chapter 10 go to http://www.emotionaldiet.com/review.html.

Chapter Eleven

The Dreaded "E" Word - Exercise

Things alter for the worse spontaneously, if they be not altered for the better designedly.   *~Francis Bacon*

Imagine this scene that probably happens somewhere every morning. Jane and Mary are good friends. They both want to be trim and healthy and they know how important exercise is to good health. At 6:00AM, the alarm goes off for both Jane and Mary, but they take very different paths.

Jane jumps up with anticipation and joy as she packs her gym bag and heads down to the nearby facility. She is filled with enthusiasm as she thinks about her workout and her friends at the gym. Mary hits the snooze alarm and rolls back over in bed. "I hate getting up in the morning", she says, "And I hate working out. This is such a drag". By the time Mary gets up, there is not enough time left to get to the fitness facility. "Maybe I'll do it after work if I have time", she thinks.

What is the difference between Jane and Mary that drives one to rush to the gym while the other avoids it like a dreaded disease? You may think that it is just the difference in personalities or maybe Jane is just a morning person. While those factors could come into play, the real answer is much simpler. Mary is focused on the process while Jane is focused on the result. When you think about the process of exercise and you see it as work, you are not motivated. This is especially true if you have negative feelings toward it. Jane is focused on the result and how good it will make her feel. She is thinking about having boundless energy, a trim, healthy body and the joy of meeting friends that share the same desire to feel healthy.

Remember the power of focus. Whatever you focus on, you get more of. If you focus on how hard this will be, you create a feeling of displeasure and you avoid doing whatever creates that feeling. When you focus on how great you will look and feel, you are drawn toward whatever will help you create that feeling.

One of my favorite people to watch is Oprah Winfrey. She often talks about her struggles with her weight and she has been such an inspiration to so many people. Recently I saw her with her trainer, Bob Greene, who has done so much to help people like Oprah change their lives in regard to good health. Oprah was talking to six people on her program and challenging them to make the commitment to change. She said that she still has to make herself get up every morning and work out, even though she hates doing it. Yes, she used the word "hate". She said, "I just hate getting up early in the morning and I hate working out. It is just something I know I have to do so I make myself do it every day". She did follow it up with, "I love the feeling I get when I am done".

As long as Oprah uses words like "I hate getting up early", and "I hate working out", it will be something she has to force herself to do. Have you ever caught yourself doing that same thing? My guess is that most people have. Let's see how we can create a feeling that helps draw us toward the actions that will give us a healthy body.

First, let's start with our words. I'm sure you knew that was coming. There are a lot of emotions connected to the word "exercise". If you are one of the people that cringe at the sound, you are not alone. I have never liked the word "exercise" because it creates in me, a feeling of something that is not going to be fun and that must be work to be of any value. Another word that creates that same feeling is "workout". Just the fact that it contains the word "work" is a turnoff for many people. For some, it can have the opposite effect. It all depends on how you internalize the word "work".

I prefer the words "move" or "energize". Your body just loves to move. When you get your body moving, so many good things start to happen. Your body is made of energy, like everything else in the universe. When you move your body, you create a charge that intensifies that energy. Remember how different your affirmations became when you added the quick movements to them? You created power affirmations, by your quick movements, which created a feeling that connected to your nervous system. You have probably heard of people who run frequently and get something called a "runner's high". This is because the movement in their body generates energy and releases endorphins that make them feel wonderful. It's no wonder they become addicted to running. They are not thinking as much about the running as they are about the great feeling they get from it. The good news is you don't have to be a runner to create that feeling. All you have to do is move.

There are many other good things that happen when you start moving more. The obvious is that you will burn more calories and remove more fat from your body. That feels good just to think about, doesn't it? You also get your heart pumping more and get more oxygen-rich blood to your muscles and vital organs. You lubricate your joints and actually make everything in your body work better. We often think that it is better for our bodies to rest more and move less. Rest is important, but so is keeping your body moving.

I once bought a car from an estate sale, which had been stored for almost three years. Because it had not been driven, there were not many miles on it and it just looked beautiful. I thought that having a low mileage car meant that it would last longer and everything would work perfectly because it hadn't been used. Wow, was I wrong! The engine leaked oil, the transmission started to have trouble shifting and the engine started to make clicking noises. My mechanic told me that the seals and gaskets had become hard and brittle because of sitting so long. Also, the oil and gas had gummed up the engine. It is harder on a car to sit than it is to be driven. The same thing is true of your body. When you sit too long, the blood will not circulate as well and your muscles and cells start to atrophy. In other words, if you don't use it, you lose it. By keeping your body moving, it will last a long time. It will also look better and feel better.

Even Thin People Can Be Fat Inside

I mentioned before that you could be at your ideal weight by eating only junk food if you limited the amount of calories you take in. Of course, you would not be healthy and you may not be as thin as you think. Being thin does not automatically mean you are not fat. Many people are at the weight they want to be according to the body mass index charts, but internally they have excess fat that is putting them at risk.

Doctors now say that the internal fat around your vital organs such as the liver, heart or pancreas could be even more dangerous than the visible fat that shows up all over the body. The scary part is that it may not even show. If your body wants to store fat in the fat cells, it looks for the easiest place to expand. Often, that is right around the middle. You could think you are healthy because you are not overweight. Meanwhile, you are at greater risk for diabetes, heart disease and other problems. Scientists believe we naturally accumulate fat around the belly first, and at some point it starts storing it somewhere else. To make things worse, a fatty liver affects your metabolism.

This means that many heavy people who are in good shape are actually healthier than those who are trim and sedentary. Remember, your goal is to be trim and healthy (and happy).

According to recent studies, people who maintain their weight through diet rather than exercise are likely to have major deposits of internal fat, even if they are otherwise thin. According to Dr. Jimmy Bell, people who are fat on the inside are essentially on the threshold of being obese. They eat too many fatty, sugary foods and exercise too little.

Dr. Bell, a professor of molecular imaging at Imperial College of London, scanned nearly 800 people with MRI machines to create "Fat Maps" showing where people store their fat. These were people with normal Body Mass Index scores of 20 to 25. What he found was that 45 percent of women and 60 percent of men actually had excessive levels of internal fat. He calls them "TOFIs" – people who are "Thin Outside, Fat Inside".

The good news is that internal fat can be burned off through exercise and improved diet. The real key is exercise. When your body uses up the available glucose in your system, it switches to the fat reserves for energy. A very restrictive diet can actually cause your body to go into starvation mode and hold on to more fat. The bottom line is, exercise not only burns fat, it makes you healthy. What could be better than that?

Exercise, rather than dieting, is the key to losing internal fat deposits.

Do What You Love and Love What You Do

As long as you think of exercise as something you "have to do" but really don't want to do, you probably will not do it. Another problem is, we usually see exercise as something we know we should do, but do not see it as a priority. After all, if we don't exercise, we can still survive. It's not like eating or sleeping.

The first thing to do is to see exercise as a priority – just like eating and sleeping. It's true that you can get by without exercising, but you will pay the price in the way you look, act and feel. Start by focusing on the outcome. Imagine yourself feeling fantastic with an abundance of energy. Imagine having a healthy glow about you and feeling as healthy as you look. Notice how people comment about how healthy you look. Notice how proud you are of yourself for taking control of your life. Notice how young and energetic you look and feel. Don't you just love that feeling?

Now imagine that you haven't exercised for awhile. Notice how tired and lethargic you feel. You want to really enjoy life to the fullest, but you just don't have the energy. You hate feeling this way, don't you? Now is the time to decide that you want to live with the energy and passion that makes your life so wonderful. All you have to do is start moving. It doesn't take much to start feeling better right now. Promise that you will move your body more each day because you deserve to feel that good.

You may be wondering how movement can give you energy. After all, it seems that exercise and movement would drain you of your energy. How can it possibly give you more energy? Well, we already talked about the emotional connection and how we feel invigorated when we combine quick movement with affirmations. Movement can also stimulate you physically. One of the best examples I can give you is a microwave oven. How is it able to cook without heat? Very simply, the microwaves excite the water molecules in the food and cause them to move which creates energy. Of course, our bodies are not capable of moving fast enough to generate heat like a microwave, but exercise does excite the cells in your body and creates energy. What if you said you want to "energize" your body? Doesn't that sound great?

In short, moving makes you feel good both physically and emotionally. When my son, Jeff, would feel emotionally tense, he would go downstairs and hit the punching bag until he released the tension. Movement and exercise will allow you to release some of the stress and tension in your life.

If you could take a magic pill that would allow you to feel healthier, look better, relieve stress, reduce tension and headaches, have more energy and live longer, would you take it? Of course you would. The great news is, you can have that magic elixir right now and it is absolutely free. Give yourself this gift of movement every day and see how great your life becomes.

One way to make exercise and movement part of your life is to combine it with something you enjoy. That way you will anchor good feelings to exercise and look forward to it every day. What do you enjoy doing? If you like spending time with friends, make it a point to walk with your friends. It doesn't have to be power walking. Even leisurely walking is good for your health and feels good.

What else could you do with your friends? How about golf, tennis or bowling? There are so many activities you can do with friends every day.

What else do you enjoy? Do you like to watch television? I have a small television, with headphones in front of my exercise bicycle. I watch many of my favorite programs as I ride. You can also just stand up and move or stretch as you watch television. Maybe you can plan your exercise around your favorite shows. What a great connection that would be.

If you enjoy music, you can walk with your portable music player or just dance around the house as you listen to music on the stereo or watch MTV.

Take a minute right now and think of some of your favorite activities and how you can enhance these activities with more movement and more pleasure.

What Kind of Exercise?

One question that people often ask is, "What kind of exercise is best?" The first answer is: whatever kind you will do. You already have an idea of how you can make a connection to what you enjoy. Now, let's get specific. If you

174

only do one thing to exercise, here it is. Every morning you should already have a ritual. You take a few minutes to relax and think about what is good in your life and what you are grateful for. This will put you in a very positive mental state. Then you practice a round of EFT for having a fantastic day and possibly another for being trim and healthy. At that point you feel really inspired. Then you do your power affirmations and you feel unstoppable. That is the time to do at least 10 minutes of some type of movement or aerobic exercise. You are starting the day emotionally charged and movement will get you physically charged. The way you start your day will have a lot to do with what kind of day you will have. Choose to make every day amazing.

Some people will question why I only suggest 10 minutes of exercise each morning. Here is the reason. Ideally, it would be better to exercise for at least 20 to 30 minutes every day. When many people think of exercising 20 or 30 minutes, they start to think about time. You ask yourself, "How will I have time to exercise that long with my busy schedule?" I've found that everyone can seem to fit 10 minutes into their schedule every morning. It may take getting up 10 minutes earlier, but it will be worth it. If you are able to spend more time exercising, that is even better. Just make it a point to give yourself that gift every morning. There is really no excuse for not spending 10 minutes to look and feel better every day. If your schedule allows more time, keep going longer. The main thing is to be consistent. Make this a part of your morning routine every day. When someone asks me if they really need to exercise every day, I answer, "No, only the days that you want to feel good!"

Here is something else you can do to maximize your time – combine your power affirmations with 10 minutes of quick movements or exercise. If you fire off those positive affirmations every morning for 10 minutes, it will intensify your feelings and you'll feel your body becoming energized by the movement. Wow! What a way to start the day!

I am actually a fan of three types of exercise. If you want to speed up your metabolism, try hitting the weights. When you increase your lean muscle mass, you automatically burn more calories, even when you are just sitting. Strength training is also good for your joints and your bones. People in their 70's and 80's will often double their strength through weight training. This means fewer injuries and greater stamina, regardless of your age. You are never too old to increase your strength with resistance training and neither are your muscles.

175

The muscle cells in your body are completely replaced, one at a time about every three or four months. That means you get new muscles two or three times every year. There is an old saying, "If you don't use it you lose it". This is especially true of your muscle cells, so let's start using them.

Aerobic exercise is probably the best for your heart and your body as far as over- all health. Your heart is actually a pump that circulates your blood through your body thousands of times every day. This pump is made up of muscles that expand and contract. The stronger your heart muscles are, the better your heart will pump blood through your body. You already knew that. But there is more to it than just moving blood around. A healthy heart is the key to a healthy body.

The third type of exercise is for flexibility and peace of mind. Yoga, Ti Chi and other far eastern types of exercise are excellent examples.

How to Put Exercise in Your Every Day Life

1) **Never Sit Through Another Commercial.** One of the biggest causes of lack of exercise is the television. The average American watches over 4 hours of TV every day. That is 4 hours of being a couch potato. The average total programming time in a half hour program is 23 minutes. That means you are sitting through 7 minutes of commercials. When the commercial comes on, jump up from your chair and do something. You can walk in place as you watch the TV, you can walk up and down the stairs a few times, you can go outside and walk around the house, or you can just walk around inside the house until the program comes back on. The key is to get up and get moving. This will speed up your metabolism, even while you are sitting. Imagine getting 15 minutes of exercise every hour while watching TV! Awesome!

2) **Park Farther Away.** When we run errands or go shopping, most of us try to park as close to the door as possible. Recently I saw a person wait almost a minute for a parking place right in front of a fitness center where they were going to work out. Does that make sense? Instead, choose a parking space at the

176

end of the aisle away from the door so you walk farther. When you are grocery shopping, don't leave your cart next to your car. Take the extra steps to return the cart to the containment area in the lot. Every step counts.

2) Use the Stairs. Some people will go to the gym and use the stair stepper and ignore the benefit that they have available every day. Walking up and down stairs will strengthen your muscles and burn calories. When you need to go up or down stairs at home, turn around and make the trip a second time. Walking stairs is great exercise. If you work several floors up, take the elevator partway and walk the last two flights. If you aren't able to walk up the stairs, but can walk down them, do that. Even going down the stairs gives you a bit of exercise and is better for you than the elevator. Walking the stairs just a few times every day will burn one pound every month.

3) Use the Inconvenient Restroom at Work. Look for a restroom that is on another floor or in another part of the building, if possible. After you've been sitting awhile, your body needs to move to improve the circulation. The extra walking will burn calories and make you more effective when you are back at your desk.

4) Dance Your Cares Away. Dancing is wonderful exercise and makes you feel good because of the music connection. If you don't have anyone to dance with, just turn on the radio and start to boogie! Let yourself go and dance to the music. We all hate to dust the furniture and do all of those chores around the house. Put on your favorite music, and dance away that dust! You can dance and move almost anywhere and anytime.

5) Pick Up Some Veggies. Canned soup or vegetables make great light hand weights. You can use them to work on upper body strength and/or range of motion. These exercises can be done one arm at a time, standing or sitting. You can do presses, curls and a number of other movements. As you get used to these movements, increase the number of repetitions or get heavier cans. You can do this while you are watching television or even at your desk at work.

6) Lift Your Feet. One easy way to exercise your legs and abs is leg lifts. This is something easy that you can do at work or at home. Sit in a steady chair and lift one leg slowly until it's parallel with the floor. Hold for a few seconds and then slowly lower it. Then repeat with the other leg. Again, as you get used to the activity, increase repetitions or try lifting both legs at once.

7) Stretch Anytime. Careful, gentle stretching feels good and is good for us. Stand with your feet shoulder width apart. Slowly bring one arm up over your head and bend at the waist in the opposite direction. Repeat the other direction. Gently bend forward at the waist. If your balance is good, put one foot on a chair and bend your knee to stretch in. These may be done by holding a chair if balance is a problem. You can also do stretches while sitting.

8) Be a Power Shopper. When you walk through the store, cruise every isle briskly and get in extra steps. You might even carry your own shopping bags for a change. That way you are not only giving your upper body a quick strength workout, but you also reduce your stress levels!

9) Flex like Arnold. Just by flexing a few times each day, you can maintain a significant amount of muscle tone. Simply flex those muscles whenever you are sitting in your car, standing at the bus stop or walking to the boss' office. Why not strike some show-off poses in your bathroom mirror while getting ready for your day?

10) Take a walk. This is my favorite. Walking is great. No expertise or equipment is required, you can do it anytime and it's free! What's more, provided you do it regularly and for long enough period of time, walking can be just as beneficial as any of the more vigorous activities (like jogging, etc). The added benefit is that it relaxes your mind and relieves stress. Walk outside if possible and connect with nature. You'll be amazed at how small your problems are and how clear your thinking becomes.

The Bottom Line

If there is anything that is the fountain of youth, it is exercise. The old saying that "if you don't use it you lose it", is so true. Moving your body invigorates every cell in your body. It builds the muscles in your heart, oxygenates your blood and pumps vital nutrients to every cell in your body. The fastest road to aging prematurely is to be dormant. If you have to choose between being heavy and in shape or being slim and out of shape, you are much better off being in shape, even with the extra weight. Keep your body moving, and it will keep going for a long time.

For a wrap-up of Chapter 11 go to http://www.emotionaldiet.com/review.html.

Chapter Twelve

Making Every Day Special

Feelings are much like waves, we can't stop them from coming but we can choose which one to surf. ~Jonatan Mårtensson

When I was in the Army, my good friend Leo would say, "Expect the worst and you'll never be disappointed". That may have seemed appropriate at the time, but what I came to realize is that you usually get just what you expect. If you expect problems, you will look for them until you find them. Haven't you known someone who was like Leo? No matter how good things are, they will keep saying, "I just know that this is not going to work". If you are not 100 percent successful, they are quick to say, "See! I told you so! I knew it wouldn't work". It is almost like they take pleasure in the failure. Actually, they probably do get a perverse form of pleasure because failure proves they were right. They keep looking for the slightest little thing to go wrong, so that they can say they were right.

Having an extraordinary life does not happen by accident. It is all about how you focus your thoughts and internalize feelings. That is why two people can have the same experience with different results. Why is it that so many famous personalities self destruct with drugs, alcohol and bizarre behavior when they seem to have everything in life they could ask for? The reason is that everyone is looking for the same thing. They want to change the way they feel. True happiness does not come from a bottle or a pill. It comes from internal feelings, and you have the ability to change those feelings anytime you want.

Daily Rituals

Humans are much like other creatures of the earth in that we are creatures of habit. Most of what we do is a conditioned response, often called a habit. Some

181

of these are done without even thinking. For example, you may put on your left shoe first every day. These habits really don't affect the way we feel. There are other things we do on a regular basis that will gradually create an outcome that determines how we act and feel about ourselves. They are the daily rituals that we feel are important, either because society or our personal desire dictate them.

For example, many people will start their day by having a cup of coffee, taking a shower, brushing their teeth, etc. It is not because they always particularly enjoy the process; it is because these are important for health or acceptable for society. The key point to remember is that we do these things every day, without questioning if they are necessary. We know they are necessary so we keep doing them.

If there is any part of your life that you want to change, you need to focus on what you want, and include daily rituals that drive your feelings and behavior. Success is not an event; it is a process like everything else. You wouldn't take one shower and say, "There! I'm clean for the rest of my life". If you want something to be part of your life, add it to your daily rituals. It is not difficult, although it does take time and commitment.

Your mind is the most powerful tool you have. The way you start your day and the way you end your day are critically important. Here is how you can create changes in any part of your life:

Start Your Day with an Attitude of Gratitude

The direction of your life is determined by your dominant thoughts. The greatest power is in the thoughts you have first thing in the morning and the last thoughts you have at night. When you first wake up, you mind is still in a relaxed state, just above the alpha state. This is perfect for giving yourself suggestions for the person you want to be. When you first get up, take 5 minutes and think about what is good in your life. Think of what you are grateful for. Then, imagine yourself as the person you intend to be. If you want more money, imagine how you would live with the money you desire. If you want to lose weight, imagine you are already the size and weight you want to be. See and feel it as though you are already exactly the way you want to be. Feel how good it feels to be that person. Notice what new behaviors you have. Notice how you go through your day as that person.

If you would like a recording of a morning session for weight loss and happiness, go to http://www.emotionaldiet.com/downloads.html.

It is 6 ½ minutes long, and it will help you get your day started the way you want.

Look at your blueprint for success to have a clear picture of what you are creating. Use your powerful imagination to create your new behavior and become the person you choose to be. Imagine yourself having already reached your goal, going through your day with confidence and ease. The life you create in your mind becomes the life you live.

Follow this exercise with a quick round of EFT. Start with this set-up:

"Even though I don't know what today will bring, I deeply and completely love and accept myself and I now choose to have an excellent day".

Now tap on the remaining meridian points. As you tap, repeat the phrase

"Excellent day"

Close your eyes, take a deep breath, hold and exhale slowly through your mouth.

Now use a few power affirmations to charge your energy system and energize yourself. You are now ready for an awesome day!

End Your Day with Excellence

When you focus your thoughts just before you go to sleep, you spend more time in rapid eye movement (REM) sleep, which internalizes the thoughts into dreams and subconscious memories. Just before you go to bed at night, think of what good things happened during the day. Relive those magic moments and enjoy them all over again. By focusing on the good events, you raise your awareness and attract more good events. If there was anything you wish you could do differently, go ahead and do it in your mind. Think of how you will do it differently next time, and see it happen in your mind. Make it as real as possible. Imagine passing up that candy and feeling so powerful. Your subconscious mind can't tell the difference between a real and a vividly imagined event. You are programming yourself for the future. An added benefit is that you will sleep better. Many restless nights are caused by worry and stress. Go to bed happy and sleep better.

Follow this with a round of EFT using the following set-up:

"Even though I can't control everything in my life, I deeply and completely love and accept myself and I now choose to have a happy life".

Now tap on the remaining meridian points. As you tap, repeat the phrase *"Happy life"*

Close your eyes, take a deep breath, hold and exhale slowly through your mouth.

Journaling for Change – Your Most Powerful Tool

One of the best tools for creating an extraordinary life with permanent change, is journaling. You don't need any special type of journal. A simple lined or unlined notebook will do. The best time to journal is late in the afternoon or evening. Many people like to journal just before going to bed. At the top of the page, write down the date and the day of the week. In your journal, write down what I call the "Magic Moments" in your life. Be sure to do this first because it puts you in a resourceful state.

We all have these magic moments going on throughout the day, but we often miss them because we are so busy. John Lennon once said, "Life is what happens when you are busy doing other things". It is easy to become so caught up in other things that we miss what is most important in our lives. These other things take your focus away and become your dominant thoughts. You begin to feel like something is missing in your life, and in reality, it is.

Your feelings are shaped by the events in your life. Often, it is not the actual events that affect you but the events you are focused on. If you are so preoccupied with your work or your problems, your attention goes there and dominates your thoughts. Now is the time to change your focus and smell the roses.

When you think of memories, your mind works somewhat like a video recorder. If you leave a tape in your recorder, tomorrow you will tape over it. When you leave your memories unattended, you tend to record over them. They are not really gone, but they are so weak that you will not be able to bring them back with your conscious mind. The key is to refocus on those events the same day. When you relive those events, you reinforce those memories and they will change the way you feel. The best time to do this is just before you go to sleep. This puts your mind at ease and you will reinforce your memories even more, as you sleep. Here is how you can fill your mind with wonderful thoughts that will last a lifetime.

Think back to the special moments of the day. Remember when someone did something for you or you did something for someone else. Remember the conversations with good friends and the smiles. Remember the hugs, the beauty of the sunrise or sunset, the flowers or the sky. As you remember each of these moments, allow yourself to go back and relive the moments, bringing the good feelings back even stronger than before. Make the colors brighter and the sounds stronger. Allow yourself to really enjoy the moments and appreciate how special your life is. Then write down one sentence to describe the memory. If you really make this strong, you will be able to look back at your journal a year from now and remember this event vividly.

Take a few minutes and write down all of the magic moments of the day and take the time to relive them. When you do this every day, two things will happen. The first is, you will begin to realize how special your life is and what is really important to you. The second thing that will happen is, you will raise your awareness of these special moments and you will begin to notice and expect them as you go through your day. Pretty soon your life becomes one long series of magic moments and you will find more happiness than you ever imagined.

Close your eyes, take a deep breath, exhale and allow your body to relax. Take another deep breath, exhale and allow your body to relax even more. Notice how easily you are able to relax and how good it feels to take time for yourself. The way you remember your experiences will determine how you feel about them. You can't change your memories, but you can change the way you remember them, by changing the structure.

The Structure of Experience

The structure of human experience is based upon a human being's five senses, or modalities of perceiving the world: what we see, hear, feel, smell and taste. Each of these modalities are composed of components called submodalities, such as color and brightness for visual, volume and tone for auditory, etc. The power of negative past events can be reduced or even eliminated by changing your own internal submodalities of those events, such as reducing the brightness and volume. Positive events can be enhanced by increasing the submodalities. You can enrich those events by making the colors and sounds stronger.

Association versus Disassociation

Another important distinction is association versus disassociation:

Association means you experience the internal representation of a past event as if you were reliving it in your own body again.

Disassociation means you experience the internal representation of a past event as if you were watching from outside your body, as another person.

Now, think back to any moments that you wish had been different. Perhaps it was the way you acted in a certain situation. Perhaps it was an opportunity that you missed.

Become disassociated from the scene. Imagine that you are seeing these events as another person, watching yourself and others in these situations. As you watch yourself, you realize that you are doing the best you can for the situation.

Appreciate yourself for that and forgive yourself and others if necessary. Think of what you can learn from this situation. Imagine how you might act differently in this situation in the future.

Then, imagine that the situation comes up again in the future, and see yourself acting the way you want with the ideal result. Allow yourself to enjoy the moment and appreciate yourself for learning and making changes. Realize that you are a special person. Slowly open your eyes, knowing that you have taken control of your life and it feels so good.

Journaling Exercise

Think of a pleasant experience you have had recently. It may have been something simple like something someone did for you or you for them. It could be a hug from a child, watching a sunset or just being with someone. Relive the moment making it brighter and stronger. Take a deep breath to anchor the feeling.

After you relive the experience, write down a few words as a reminder phrase.

Think of something that happened recently that you wish had turned out differently. Go through the disassociation/association exercise and write down your new behavior. Example: I always remain calm when driving in traffic.

The Law of Attraction

A lot has been written lately about the law of attraction. The basic concept is that you can attract anything into your life that you want just by thinking about it. The more you think about it and the more feeling you put into your thoughts, the stronger the attraction becomes. The down side is that if you have something in your life that you don't want or you are not happy about, it is because you attracted it with your thoughts. Some of it may seem a bit hard to accept when you think of people living in poverty or sickness. Did they really bring that on themselves?

The law of attraction is real and it does exist. At the same time, there is more to it than just sitting still and wishing for your life to be perfect. Wishing is the starting point but not the ending point.

This is where I differ from some people that claim the law of attraction will bring them everything they want. It is like each of us is a magnet just waiting to attract what we want by rubbing Aladdin's magic lamp and waiting for our wishes to be granted. I believe that it is the other way around. I think whatever we want is the magnet and we are the steel that is attracted to it.

I mentioned before that we are drawn toward whatever we focus on. When you focus on what you want, magical things can happen. You will see things you never saw before. It may be that they were always there but now you finally see them for the first time. There is a part of your brain called the reticular activating system. Basically, it helps you raise your awareness of possibilities and opportunities that you never realized even existed.

When you focus your attention on anything, either good or bad, you will attract more of it. Or to be more specific, you will be attracted to it. If you want happiness, you have to look for it. If you want good health, you have to look for it. If you want a better relationship, you have to look for it. If you expect good things, you will find them. If you expect bad things, you will find them.

I mentioned this in one of my seminars and one person said, "Well! That explains everything!" We all looked at her for a further explanation. She said that her best friend had been in an abusive relationship for several years. When the relationship finally ended, she thought she would find happiness at last. Within a few months, she was in another abusive relationship. This person went on to say that she thought it was just an unfortunate coincidence until she repeated the same pattern over and over until she had five abusive relationships in a row. At that point, she was pretty sure the problem was something she was doing.

Even though she wanted a good relationship, her mind was constantly on the bad relationships she had been in before. She focused on what she didn't want and in return, she got just what she focused on. The reason she got into her first bad relationship was because her father had been abusive. To her, this was normal behavior. I don't mean that she consciously thought this was normal or right. In her subconscious mind, she connected this behavior to what she had grown up with and was used to experiencing.

If you are unhappy with any part of your life right now, you have the power to change. It all starts with the law of attraction. If you want a better relationship, you have to identify what kind of a relationship you want. What attributes would you like in the other person? What activities would you like to spend time doing? What would your life be like? You have to be clear on what you want before you can attract it. At the beginning of this book, you created a blueprint for success. This was the key to clearly defining the person you intended to be. You can use the same process to create changes in any part of your life. If you want more money, friends, happiness or anything else, you must decide exactly what you want and have a clear vision. As you focus on what you want, notice the world around you. You will find that doors will open for you and possibilities will appear.

To really apply the law of attraction, you need to do more than dream and visualize your outcome. The key to success is to activate your feelings. When you allow yourself to imagine what you want as though it has already happened and feel as though you have already achieved it, your whole perspective will change. You will change your beliefs and actions to become the kind of person that can achieve those dreams.

The second part of the law of attraction is the most important part and the one that is talked about the least. ACTION! When those doors open for you, (and they will open), you have to go through the doors. Think of all the opportunities you have had in your life that you missed because you didn't act on them when you had the chance. Now decide that you will focus on what you want and look for new opportunities to appear. When opportunity knocks on your door, for gosh sakes...answer it! Go through that door and find the happiness you deserve. Don't wait for happiness to come to you. Happiness is too busy spending time with the people that are looking for it. Decide what you want, have a clear vision, engage your feelings and watch for the doors to open.

Avoid Negative People

Negative people are like a plague. They are not satisfied to feel bad by themselves. They feel this need to spread their negative feelings to everyone around them. They can have a very damaging effect on the entire group of people they interact with. These effects can be physical, as well as emotional. Since your emotions directly affect your immune system, you owe it to yourself to feel good every day. Life is meant to be enjoyed, and every day you spend feeling down is like throwing away a day of your life. It is important to protect yourself from the negative people and your own negative feelings.

Nothing is totally good or bad – it is all in your perspective. It's like the glass that is half empty or half full. It is how you look at it. The best technique for altering your perspective is called *reframing*. Basically you look at any situation and reframe it in a different light. For example, if you feel you have to pay too much in taxes, you could reframe that by saying, "Isn't it great that I made this much money". Another reframe might be, "Isn't it great that I have a job to pay taxes". If you are stuck in traffic you might think to yourself, "Isn't it great that I have a car to drive".

One of my favorite questions (thanks to Tony Robbins) to ask about any situation is, "What is good about this?" Another one is, "What can I learn from this? How can I use this to make me a better person?"

Since it is not always possible to keep the negative people out of your life, here is the best method I know of for staying up, when they are trying to bring you down. The most important thing you can do is to get in the last word. Always cover a negative statement with a positive one. The last thing you hear tends to stay in your mind. It's kind of like that song that you just keep hearing over and over again.

Make sure the last thing you hear (and that others hear) is positive. If someone says something negative, say something positive about the same thing. You don't have to be argumentative and you can even agree with them while reframing. This week I was walking out of a business and the person next to me said, "Wow! This heat and humidity is just miserable." I looked back at him and replied, "Well, at least we don't have to shovel it and I've never gotten stuck in humidity!" You will usually change the other person's emotional state and sometimes you will even get a laugh. When that happens, you know that they realize that things are not so bad and in fact, they are really pretty good.

Celebrate Success

Earlier in the book I suggested making your happiness unconditional. Too often we say things like, "When I lose 20 pounds, then I'll be happy" or "When I get a better job, I'll be happy". To your subconscious mind that becomes, "I'll have to be unhappy until I reach my goal". Don't let your happiness depend on something else happening. Let your happiness be internally driven instead of externally driven. You can't control what happens to the rest of the world or how someone else will act. You can control how you feel. In fact, that is just about the only thing in your life that you can control. Unfortunately, most of us wait for someone or something else to make us feel better. The problem with that is the other person or situation may not turn out to be the way we imagined or wanted, and we feel disappointed.

I remember reading an article in the paper, about a seventy one year old Chicago man who was attempting to become the oldest man to climb Mount Everest. What really caught my eye was that they said he "failed in his two previous attempts, the last one being two years ago when he came within 300 feet of the summit". Three hundred feet! That is the length of a football field! He was that close to the highest point in the world, and they said he failed because they focused on the 300 feet he didn't climb and they ignored the 28,729 feet that he did climb.

So often we define success as reaching a goal. Having a goal is nice because it keeps us focused on where we want to go. The problem happens when you decide that success depends on whether or not you reach that goal. For so many people, falling short of their goal is failure. The only real failure is to not try. As long as you try something, you will always get a result. That is success. Give yourself credit for making the effort and then ask how you can do it differently next time. Be sure to enjoy the experience along the way. If your goal is to become 20 pounds thinner and you stop at 15, feel proud of where you are and be happy with the progress you have made.

Live in the Moment

Recently, someone asked me recently how I handle stress. I told them that I don't do stress. What I mean by that is that stress is really internal. We all create our own stress by our thoughts. It is not what happens to us that creates the stress, it is how we react to it.

If you are feeling stress right now, it is probably because you are thinking about something that hasn't happened and are worrying about how it might turn out. The other possibility, is that you are thinking about the past and wondering why things happened as they did or why something is not the same as it was. If you are not in physical pain, the only thing keeping you from feeling good at this moment, is your focus.

I worked with one person who was clinically depressed and had not had any relief after ten years of working with psychologists and psychiatrists. I asked him to think of something he really enjoyed and he said skiing. I said that was a great example of using his focus. When he was skiing, he had to focus on the present moment. He had no time to worry about the past or the future when he was flying down a mountain at sixty miles per hour. By focusing on the joy of the moment, he was able to be free of his depression.

Most people focus on the future and worry about what might go wrong. Others think about what did go wrong in the past and keep reliving those negative events. This creates feelings of sadness and regret. If you live in the moment and focus on what is good in your life right now, you will feel the joy of life.

Forgive Yourself and Others

Have you ever done something in your life that you regret? Who hasn't? Has someone else ever done something that you didn't like? That has happened to everyone. We all have these painful memories that we hang on to, wishing that they hadn't happened. Well, life happens. We are going to do things we regret and other people are going to let us down. It is part of life. One of the most beneficial ways to feel better is to let go of these negative feelings. Holding on to them will only make you bitter. Your life is too precious to waste even one moment feeling bad, when you can choose to feel good.

Think of someone who has done something in the past to hurt you. As you do this, imagine that they are becoming very small – much smaller than you. Realize that they may be doing the best they can, or they may have had an unhappy childhood or bad relationships. Your first reaction may be to say, "Well, that's not my fault". This is no time to look for fault. It is a time to try to understand. Even if that is hard for you to do, imagine that person is there now and tell them that you forgive them. Many people will say that they don't want to forgive someone for the pain and hurt they caused. Realize this; forgiveness is not a gift you give to others, it is a gift you give to yourself. It is time to let go of the pain, and free yourself from the bonds of the past. Try saying it out loud and really feel the forgiveness coming to life.

Now, think of a time when you hurt someone or felt like you disappointed someone including yourself. You'll probably still feel the pain. Often we will mask the pain by putting the blame somewhere else. No one likes to feel bad about them self. Now, realize that you can't change the past. What you can do is learn from the past and forgive yourself for your actions. Say it out loud with feelings. If you still feel some negative emotions, use EFT to release those feelings:

Set Up
"Even though I still have some painful feelings when I think about

_____,

I deeply and completely accept myself and I now choose to let go of these feelings".

Reminder – alternate between the two

These feelings about _____.

I now choose to forgive myself / someone else for _____.

Avoid Putting Negative Labels on Yourself

I recently worked with someone who first described herself as "Morbidly Obese". I know there is a medical definition for this term. According to the National Institutes of Health, a person is considered "obese" when he or she weighs 20 percent or more than his or her ideal body weight. At that point, the person's weight poses a real health risk. Obesity becomes "morbid" when it significantly increases the risk of one or more obesity-related health conditions or serious diseases. Morbid obesity—sometimes called "clinically severe obesity"—is defined as being 100 lbs. or more over ideal body weight or having a Body Mass Index (BMI) of 40 or higher.

It is important to recognize where you are and to not be blind to reality. The problem with labels is that people often label themselves and then their subconscious mind does everything possible to make sure their actions and behaviors match that identity. This is not only true of your body; it is true of any part of your life.

Have you ever forgotten something? Sure, we all have. Does that mean you are forgetful? Only if you decide you are. If you do, you will notice that you become more forgetful all the time because you now identify with that behavior and that label.

I worked with a young woman who was diagnosed as being "clinically depressed". She had spent several years working with psychologists and psychiatrists with no solution. I asked her when she felt these feelings of depression and she said, "All of the time". Then she reminded me that she was "clinically depressed". I realized that she identified with her behavior and had become exactly what her doctors told her she was. I'm not suggesting that she was not dealing with depression – only that she would have a difficult time changing her feelings as long as she held on to that label.

194

What are some labels you have put on yourself? Have you ever said you were fat? How about weak or a failure? Have you ever called yourself stupid or boring or any one of a million labels you could put on yourself? Now is the time to change the way you see yourself.

Realize that you are not your behavior or your label. You are not fat; you are a wonderful person who has extra weight on your body. You are not stupid; you are an intelligent person that needs a better organizing system. You are not a failure; you are an amazing person who is constantly looking for the key to success.

Here is a great exercise that is sure to put a smile on your face and start your day the right way. When you get up in the morning, look in the mirror and tell yourself how fantastic you are. Tell yourself how much you have learned and all of the great things you have done. Then tell yourself how much you love yourself and forgive yourself for anything you may feel bad about. I know how silly this sounds, especially when you really imagine doing this. In fact, most people say it does feel a bit silly the first time they do it. Then they realize they are giving themselves a wonderful gift, and it becomes part of their daily routine. Give it a try tomorrow morning (or, if you just can't wait, do it right now).

Identifying What is Most Important to You

The main reason that people are not happy or fulfilled is because they are not aligned with their values. I talked to a man recently who was telling me about how his job was just burning him out. No matter how far up the corporate ladder he climbed, it never seemed to really satisfy him. It was like the bar was being raised just as he was reaching it. The real problem was that he was the one that kept raising the bar.

I asked him why he kept trying to go higher. What was it he really wanted? He had never thought about it before. Then I asked him if he was truly happy. He thought about it for a moment and said, "No.......no, I'm not happy. Then I asked him, "What would make you happy?"

The way to find out what makes you happy is to identify what is really important to you and why. You may find that you are chasing an illusion that someone else has created. The world is full of ads and television programs that picture the life of your dreams. The question is; is it really your dream?

When I asked the businessman to identify what was most important to him, he replied, "My family! That's why I work 12 hours a day!" Then I asked him the most important question of all. Are you spending your time on the things that matter most to you? He realized that what gave him the most joy was where he was spending the least amount of time. The time he did have at home was spent doing the necessary chores with little quality time for the people he loved.

Where are you spending your time? Is it on the things that are most important to you? If health is one of your values (at this point, it had better be), did you spend at least as much time exercising as you did watching television? Are you missing the real joy in your life because you have never really taken the time to identify what is most important to you? Are you following your dreams or following your fears?

Make a list of what is most important to you right now. There is no right amount of values on the list. It is what is right for you. Then take a look at the past week or month and see how much time you have spent on what matters to you the most. When you spend time on what matters most to you, you will feel fulfilled.

My most important values are:

(Here are just a few ideas to start your thinking.)

love	friendship	family
peace	stability	relationships
joy	wisdom	freedom
happiness	knowledge	comfort
independence	serenity	sex
security	passion	intimacy
adventure	health	faith
fitness	courage	giving

My most important values are:

What is most important to you in your life?

_____

_____

_____

_____

_____

_____

_____

_____

_____

_____

_____

_____

_____

_____

Continue Your Journey

Even though you have reached the end of this book, you have really just begun your journey. You now have the tools to change almost anything in your life. Remember that this is not a one-time process. It takes repetition and emotion to create the life you desire. A setback can be a setup for success. Learn from every experience. When you do that, there are no failures.

Another suggestion is to involve your friends. One of the key reasons that groups like Weight Watchers are successful is because of the group support. Teach these techniques to others and get them involved as well. Plan a group meeting every week or two and support each other. Often, you will gain insight from others that you can't see yourself.

Occasionally, I will teach a four week session on these techniques at the local community college. It is interesting to see how people love to share their success stories as the weeks go on. In return, the others will find inspiration and strength from hearing of this success. The groups often take on a life of their own and continue to meet and support each other. When I present healthy living seminars for corporations, the last thing I do is organize the group to continue their meetings.

Also, continue learning new information about health and happiness. The more you understand about how your body and emotions work, the better you are at creating your ideal healthy life. I have included a list of some of my favorite books on www.emotionaldiet.com.

At the end of this book I have included a daily checklist to help you continue your journey. There is also a bonus section with 25 ways to keep yourself trim, healthy and happy.

I wish you all of the success in the world.

Bill Cashell

For a wrap-up of Chapter 12 go to http://www.emotionaldiet.com/review.html.

25 Simple Steps to Keep Yourself Trim, Healthy & Happy

1. Eliminate Mindless (unconscious) Eating - avoid multi-tasking
Studies show that people who eat while engaged in another activity will eat more than if they are just eating. If you are watching television, talking on the phone or doing any other activity that occupies your mind, it is so easy to just keep eating without realizing it. When the commercial comes on, you look down and say, "Who ate all of my popcorn?"

2. Go to Bed With an Empty Stomach
This doesn't mean you have to be starving at night. When you go to bed on a full stomach, your body is busy digesting and you don't sleep as well. Try to eat smaller evening meals, and stop eating at least 3 hours before bedtime.

3. Go to Bed Happy
Before you go to bed, use EFT, journaling or any other technique to go to sleep in a good frame of mind. When you go to bed worrying, your sleep is not as deep or restful, and your stress level goes up.

4. Eat Breakfast
When you go to sleep at night, your body slows down. This includes your metabolism, which will stay slow until it has a reason to speed up. When you eat breakfast, it jump-starts your metabolism and you start burning calories faster. A healthy breakfast will also help you think better. University studies have shown that students who eat a healthy breakfast of complex carbohydrates average 25% better on tests. And here is one more benefit: people who eat a healthy breakfast have less illness – as much as 40% less. A breakfast of oatmeal and blueberries will clear your arteries and boost your immune system.

5. Enjoy the Feeling of an Empty Stomach

Most people have created an association of pleasure with having a full stomach. This can cause us to eat even when we are not hungry. If you associate the feeling of pleasure to having an empty stomach, you can lose that desire to over- eat.

6. Take Three Deep Breaths Before Eating

You should already be doing deep power breathing three times per day. This is a great way to include your deep breathing, plus the relaxation of the deep breathing will help relieve any tension that may be triggering overeating.

7. Avoid the White Stuff

When choosing bread or grain products, be sure to look for the words "Whole Grain" on the label. Whole grain bread is rich in fiber and is slower digesting than white bread. If it says "Whole Wheat", that does not mean it is whole grain. It is still a better choice than anything made with highly processed white flour. If it says "enriched", "unbleached", or "unbromated", it is still made with white flour. The best bet is to look for "100% Whole Grain". Products can be advertised as whole grain even if only part of it is whole grain.

8. Plan Meals Around Fruits and Vegetables

Most people plan their menu by starting with the meat and desserts, and then use the fruits and vegetables as fillers. When you begin with the fruits and vegetables, it causes you to focus more on the healthy foods for menu planning.

9. Never Eat From the Source

When eating anything that comes in a package, always put the amount you want to eat in a bowl or on a plate. When you eat from the package, you don't know how much you are eating and it is easy to overeat without noticing.

10. Eat Like the French

French people enjoy their food without the weight problems Americans have. They avoid gulping down their food or eating in front of a TV. The French like to eat slowly and savor their food. Dining is a pleasurable experience created by enjoying the taste and not being concerned by the amount.

11. Exercise Early

When you first get up in the morning, your body is low on available carbohydrates. If you exercise in the morning before eating, it forces the body to burn fat for energy. It also jump-starts your metabolism.

12. Think Blue

The color of your surroundings can affect your mood and also your appetite. For example, red and yellow have been shown to stimulate your appetite. Have you ever noticed what colors are used by McDonald's and Burger King? The best color to calm your appetite is blue. If you put your food on a blue plate, it will calm your appetite and you will feel less anxiety. You might even consider adding a touch of blue to your dining room and kitchen.

13. Put on Some Soothing Music

Visual cues are not the only sensory connections that affect the way we eat. If you listen to lively upbeat music, it can put you in a great mood. It can also trigger a feeling of excitement that can stimulate your appetite and cause you to eat faster. Quiet, soothing music will create a calming effect on your nervous system causing you to relax and eat slower.

14. Eat Slowly.

You probably already know that when you eat too fast, your brain does not get the message that you are full until it is too late and you have overeaten. New research shows that eating too fast can also affect the way your body processes food. When the food comes too fast, the digestive system tends to shut down and store the remaining food for later use. Guess how it stores this excess food? If you guessed fat, give yourself a star and then slow down.

15. Use a Smaller Plate

This seems too simple and some people dismiss how effective it can be. Studies have shown that people who are inclined to eat everything on their plate will do the same thing no matter what size plate they have. Even more interesting is that people who tend to stop after eating half the food on their plate will do the same thing no matter what size plate they have. Even when you consciously think about the fact that you have less food with a smaller plate, you still have to make the effort to go back and refill the plate to have more. The bottom line is this; if it is in front of you, you are more likely to keep eating than if you had to get up to get more.

16. The Handy Way to Measure Food
The average stomach is about one liter. That is about the size of your fist. That same stomach has the ability to expand about four times its size. An easy way to measure is to look at your food and see if it is larger than your fist. If the food is flat on the plate, use your open hand to measure.

17. Avoiding the Traps When You Go Out to Eat
You probably think that eating out is a recipe for failure. You do need to be careful, but it can be done. Here are the facts, courtesy of Web MD:

Most restaurants brush butter or oil on dishes like steak, chicken, and fajitas to improve their appearance. So ask for a no-butter meal. Also, remember to hold the mayo and the cheese on all dishes.

Pull the skin from your chicken and blot the oil from your pizza with a napkin. It might not be the best manners, but it can save hundreds of calories and saturated fat.

Watch your portion sizes. Ask for a doggie bag with your meal and immediately put half of it away. In addition, take one slice of bread and give the basket back to the server. To eliminate the temptation to keep nibbling on what's left on your plate when you've had enough, douse the scraps with salt, or pour on the hot sauce. By limiting portion size and asking the chef to go light, you can have a healthy meal and enjoy your evening.

18. Add Low-Fat Dairy with Calcium to Your Meals
New studies show that adding calcium-rich dairy to your meals can have a big effect on how much fat your body retains. These foods actually bind with the fat in your digestive system and prevent much of it from being absorbed by your body. In fact, as much as 50 percent of the fat you eat can be eliminated

this way. This doesn't mean you should go out and start eating cheesecake by the pound. Calories and fat still matter.

19. Eat Yogurt

One of the best choices of dairy calcium is yogurt because it is low in fat and has the added benefit of live cultures. Active cultures are the good bacteria that aid intestinal health and combat bad bacteria. Three servings of yogurt per week have been shown to boost the immune system.

20. Go Nuts

Eat a small handful of nuts about twenty minutes before your meal. The nuts provide the healthy fats and protein that help curb your appetite. The healthy fats will also help your body absorb fat-soluble vitamins from your salad and green vegetables. The best are almonds and walnuts. Be sure to stop after a handful (about a half-dozen walnuts) because nuts are higher in calories.

21. Keep Your Food on the Right Side

Here is something you probably haven't thought of before. The right side of your brain is the emotional, creative side. The left side is the logical, thinking side. Also, the right side of your brain controls the left side of your body and the left side of your brain controls the right side of your body. That means that when you look at something on your left side, you are using the right (emotional) side of your brain. Those emotion desires will become even stronger. Move the food to the right side so that you see it with the left (logical) side of your brain. I'm not saying that you will never eat anything that is on your right side, it is just lowering the emotional connection as much as possible.

22. Get Enough Sleep

Studies show that people that are tired because of lack of sleep will often try to stimulate their bodies with food instead of rest. This leads to extra calories in place of what your body really needs, which is rest. On the average, sleep deprived people eat 300 to 400 more calories per day. For the people that spend the whole week in a tired state, this could add one to two pounds in a month. There is another downside to sleep deprivation. When you don't get enough rest, your immune system is weakened. This will leave you more susceptible to colds, flu and almost all other illnesses. Pay attention to your body and how you feel. When you notice you are tired, take a short nap or at least close your eyes and relax for a few minutes. This will help you feel better without adding more calories.

23. Treat Yourself Like a Pet.

If you are not a pet owner, just imagine that you are. Would you keep your pet up late at night, wake it up early, give it a donut and coffee for breakfast, make it do something stressful all day, keep it inside without exercise, feed it tacos and beer for dinner and expect it to be happy and healthy? The fact is, most people take better care of their pets than they do themselves. The next time you are inclined to eat some unhealthy food, ask yourself, "Would I feed this to my pet?"

24. Drink More Water

It is estimated that seventy five percent of Americans are chronically dehydrated. In many people, the thirst mechanism is so weak that it is often mistaken for hunger. Even mild dehydration will slow down your metabolism and lack of water is the number one cause of daytime fatigue. According to a study at the University of Washington, one glass of water late in the evening was able to stop hunger pangs for almost all dieters in the study. As far as health benefits, drinking 8 glasses of water daily decreases the risk of colon cancer, breast cancer, and bladder cancer.

25. To Weigh Less, Eat More

Two new Penn State studies show that people who eat a healthy, low-fat, low-calorie-dense diet that includes more water-rich foods, such as fruits and vegetables, consume more food, but weigh less than people who eat a more calorie-dense diet. Water-rich foods are also a great way to keep your energy, health and vitality high.

Final Thoughts

As I sit here struggling for the right words to express my feelings, I am at a loss. It has been exactly four weeks since I lost my son Jeff, and the pain is still as strong as ever. I always thought that the most painful experience a parent could ever go through is the loss of a child. At this point, I am convinced that it is true for me.

Last year Jeff experienced anxiety and panic attacks. They became so severe that he ended up going to a crisis center for help. We didn't know about it until he called us from the center. The doctors there put him on prescription drugs to control the anxiety and referred him to a psychiatrist. Instead of helping him with his emotional problems, they just kept upping the dosage of these highly addictive drugs, without warning him of the awful side effects. The withdrawal from some of these drugs can take as long as two years, with a recommended reduction of no more than two percent per week.

Jeff was always very health conscious and loved being in good shape. He hated being on the drugs and wanted off of them as soon as possible. One psychiatrist put him on a very aggressive program to reduce them by ten percent each week. It turned out to be more than he could handle and he ran out before his next scheduled appointment. The doctor would not give him a refill without seeing him, and could not see him before the scheduled appointment. By that time, Jeff had been without the drugs for three days and felt so bad he couldn't make the appointment. It hurt so much to see him like that and we felt so helpless.

Jeff decided that he would just fight his way through the withdrawal no matter how long and painful it was. Aspirin and over the counter pain medication did not help at all. We tried everything we could to help him through the pain. I can still hear the sound of him moaning as I felt so helpless. We begged him to get help, but Jeff had his mind made up. When he started something, he wouldn't give up.

This went on for three weeks before we thought the pain might be easing a bit. Then it came back again, just as strong. What we didn't know was that he had internal bleeding. When we finally realized that something was seriously wrong, it was too late.

The past four weeks have been a constant flood of emotions – grief, pain, guilt, remorse and that awful feeling of loss. The first few days were the worst days of my life. Nothing I did would ease the painful feelings. I knew all of the techniques for releasing negative emotions and changing my thoughts, but nothing seemed to work. I realized that it wasn't the techniques. It was the fact that I didn't want to let the feelings go.

I thought back to a couple that had come to me a few months before for weight issues. They said they both started to gain weight and develop bad habits seven years before. I asked what was happening in their lives at that time, and they both looked at each other. Then they told me of the passing of their teenage daughter. We spent the next three weeks releasing the pain, guilt and negative emotions that they had held on to for seven years. After that, they lost their emotional need to eat.

My wife, Kathy, suggested that perhaps they had been put into my life to teach us how to deal with this pain. I knew that I didn't want to go through seven years of depression as they had. I also knew that I wasn't ready or willing to let go of these feelings. Then I thought of a process called the Sedona Method. The process basically has you ask a series of questions, such as: Can I embrace this feeling? If not, can I let go of it? If not now, when? This basically allows you to examine your feelings and decide how long you need to hold them before letting go. This allows you to acknowledge the feelings as necessary, but temporary. Every day I ask myself if I can let go today, and every day I let go of a little more.

We had many friends bring over cakes, cookies, and other food that I normally do not even care for. I asked Kathy what we would do with all of this food, and she said, "It would be a shame to throw it away after such caring friends made it for us. I looked at the food and felt the love and concern they had for us. That association was all it took to start an eating binge. I didn't stop until all of the food was gone. After all I've learned, even I am not immune to emotional eating.

As the days have gone by, I have returned to normal eating again. I refuse to feel guilty about eating like that and I refuse to be trapped by that behavior. There are times we may have to find any way we can to cope with our problems, but they don't have to be permanent behavior patterns.

The same techniques outlined in this book are what I have used to cope with my challenging situation. Life is not always smooth and easy. There are bumps in the road of life. Just remember that a setback is not a failure. I remember a Japanese phrase describing the key to success. It was simply, "fall down seven times; get up eight". If you have a setback, it is an opportunity for a comeback. The game isn't over until you say it is. If you refuse to give up, you will be successful.

So often in these pages, I mentioned that we are drawn toward whatever we focus on. This is probably the key to everything we do. We decided that we would not focus on what we lost, but rather on what we received. Instead of a funeral, we had a celebration of life. Instead of a coffin, we had a picture board. At the service, his brothers talked about all of the fun Jeff had and how he touched so many people. His uncle and cousin talked about the great times with Jeff and told stories that made us laugh. Then we watched a video of Jeff as he went through different stages of life.

We created a celebration of life card for the service with a collage of photos of Jeff and his family. He was smiling in every one. That is how we want to remember him. We could have chosen not to have children and been spared this pain, but then we would have missed the joy of having Jeff in our lives. So much of finding happiness in life is choosing to focus on what is good.

I tell you this story because there will be times in your life when you do face challenges. Look to yourself for joy, instead of trying to find it in food. When you look for happiness, you will find it.

We put our feelings on the back of Jeff's celebration of life card. You will find that on the next page. I hope you can find some inspiration for your life in these words.

What would you tell God?

What if God said.......

I'll give you a son. But you can only have him for 28 years.

He will give you great challenges...and great joy.

I will make him curious, and difficult at times. There will be times when he will test you to your limit. And then he will love you with all of his heart.

Life will not always be easy for him or for you. But everything you go through, you will go through together. You will laugh and you will cry. But you will always be proud to call him your son.

What would you tell God?

Dear God,

We would be honored to accept your wondrous gift.

We will name him Jeff, and we will love and cherish every moment we have with him.

We will be the best parents we can be and we will always be there for him. He will be loved by his family and friends.

And when you come to take him back, we will wish we could have had more time. But we will know that we were blessed.

And we will feel sadness that it is time for him to go. But most of all, we will feel joy for his life that touched so many.

And we will celebrate the gift of 28 years with him.

> Thank you,
> Bill & Kathy

Daily Checklist

Morning: 5 minutes

Find a relaxing place, close your eyes and think about what is good in your life. Then focus on the "you" that you are becoming. Imagine yourself going through your day with your healthy new habits. Use EFT to having a great day.

Take 10 deep power breaths followed by E-Motional affirmations.

Afternoon / evening: 20 minutes

Listen to your CD or use your self-hypnosis script

Use EFT for Trim and Healthy

Before bed: 10 minutes

Journaling:

- What was good about today? Anchor your good feelings
- What behavior would I like to change? (If any)
- Is there anyone I need to forgive (including myself)
- What did I eat today? Goal: 50% Healthy, 80% rating of 5 and above. How much water did I drink?
- Take 10 deep power breaths
- Use EFT for Happy Life (or anything else you choose)

Anytime during the day:

Practice E-Motional affirmations (E + M = E-Motion) at any time, such as driving your car, after self-hypnosis or anytime you want to add good feelings to your day.

Before you eat:

- Ask yourself if you are really hungry
- Close your eyes, take a deep breath, as you exhale imagine yourself slim and healthy. Make a powerful gesture and feel the E-Motion.
- Rate your food – 1 through 10. Make sure half of your meal is in the Healthy Group. Make sure that 80% has a value of 5 or above.
- Eat slowly (mindful eating)

Emotional desire to eat:

- Focus on what you will gain by not eating and what you will lose by eating
- Use your "feel good" anchor to give you the feeling that you think the food will give you
- Use EFT for cravings
- Use EFT for driving emotion

Date _____ **Journaling** Day _____

What were the special moments today? Relive them and anchor the feelings.

What did you learn today that will make your life better?

Think of anything you would like to do differently. See the old behavior disassociated. Write your new behavior. See the new behavior. Then, live the new behavior.

Write down what you ate today. Assign a point value.
Goal: 50% healthy, 80% 5 or above.

If you ate an excess of unhealthy foods, use your imagination to make them less attractive and make healthy foods more attractive.

Recommended Reading

Am I Hungry? What to Do When Diets Don't Work
by Michelle May, Lisa Galper & Janet Carr

Ask and It Is Given: Learning to Manifest Your Desires
by Esther Hicks & Jerry Hicks

The Best Life Diet Revised and Updated
by Bob Greene

The EFT Manual (EFT: Emotional Freedom Techniques)
by Gary Craig

The End of Diets: Healing Emotional Hunger
by Dilia de la Altagracia

Eat This, Not That! Thousands of Simple Food Swaps that Can Save You
10, 20, 30 Pounds--or More!
by David Zinczenko and Matt Goulding

Get the Life You Want: The Secrets to Quick and Lasting Life Change with
Neuro-Linguistic Programming
by Richard Bandler

Inspiration: Your Ultimate Calling
by Wayne W. Dyer

Keep it Off: Use the Power of Self-Hypnosis to Lose Weight Now
by Brian Alman

Love, Medicine and Miracles: Lessons Learned about Self-Healing from a
Surgeon's Experience with Exceptional Patients
by Bernie S. Siegel

The Promise of Energy Psychology: Revolutionary Tools for Dramatic Personal
Change
by David Feinstein, Donna Eden and Gary Craig

Spontaneous Healing : How to Discover and Embrace Your Body's Natural Ability
to Maintain and Heal Itself
by Andrew Weil

You Can Heal Your Life
by Louise L. Hay

YOU: The Owner's Manual: An Insider's Guide to the Body that Will Make You
Healthier and Younger
by Michael F. Roizen & Mehmet Oz

You: On A Diet: The Owner's Manual for Waist Management
by Mehmet C. Oz & Michael F. Roizen

You: Staying Young: The Owner's Manual for Extending Your Warranty
by Michael F. Roizen & Mehmet C. Oz

You'll See It When You Believe It
by Wayne W. Dyer

Younger Next Year: Live Strong, Fit, and Sexy—Until You're 80 and Beyond
by Chris Crowley & Henry S. Lodge, M.D

Your Miracle Brain
by Jean Carper

About the Author

Bill Cashell is an award-winning speaker, author and seminar leader. He is a leading expert on changing behavior, and has helped hundreds of people lose weight and break free from emotional eating.

Bill is an expert in personal development and human potential, and is certified in Hypnotherapy, Neuro Linguistic Programming and Emotional Freedom Techniques. He works with individuals, organizations and businesses to create positive changes in their lives and organizations. His presentations are inspiring, informative and will leave your listeners wanting more.

- Do you have a company meeting?
- Does your organization have an annual event?
- Do you attend a conference or convention that could benefit from one of Bill's dynamic presentations?

If you would like a memorable speaker for your next event or a workshop for your group or organization, contact Bill at bill@emotionaldiet.com or visit the websites at www.BillCashell.com or www.EmotionalDiet.com.

To see additional books and programs by Bill, visit www.BillCashell.com.

Be happy and healthy.

Bill

Quick Order Form

Order additional copies of this book for the discounted rate of only $15 each. You can have them signed and personalized at no extra cost.

Volume discounts are available for large orders. Email your requests to orders@fountainhillpublishing.com.

Easy online orders at www.FountainHillPublishing.com.

☐ The Emotional Diet, includes self hypnosis CD $15

☐ The Emotional Diet Audio Program on CD, includes self hypnosis and visualization sessions $37

☐ The Emotional Diet Seminar on DVD, includes audio self hypnosis and visualization sessions $57

Please send me more FREE information on:

☐ Other books   ☐ Speaking/Seminars   ☐ Consulting

Name: _____

Address: _____

City: _____ State: _____ Zip: _____

Email address: _____

Regular Shipping: $2.50 first item, $1.00 for each additional item.

Priority Shipping: $4.50 first item, $2.00 for each additional item.

Sales Tax: Please add 5.5% for products shipped to Nebraska addresses.

6118637R0

Made in the USA
Lexington, KY
19 July 2010